Georgia J. Anetzberger, PhD, ACSW. LISW
Editor

The Clinical Management of Elder Abuse

The Clinical Management of Elder Abuse has been co-published simultaneously as *Clinical Gerontologist*, Volume 28, Numbers 1/2 2005.

Pre-publication REVIEWS, COMMENTARIES, EVALUATIONS . . .

"PROVIDES A SOUND, CASE-BASED APPROACH to understanding elder abuse and the complexity that clinicians face when caring for elderly patients who suffer from any type of mistreatment. It will be ESPECIALLY USEFUL TO SOCIAL WORKERS IN HEALTH CARE SETTINGS as they evaluate and create care plans for the myriad of forms for elder mistreatment. THE LEGAL CHAPTER IS PARTICULARLY STRONG and will serve as a ready guide for health care workers who strive to meet the needs of these victims. The case studies are useful, not only for understanding the phenomenon, but also for teaching others who are striving to grasp the complexities of elder mistreatment."

Terry Fulmer, PhD, RN, FAAN
Head,
Division of Nursing,
New York University

More pre-publication
REVIEWS, COMMENTARIES, EVALUATIONS . . .

"THIS EXCELLENT, GROUND-BREAKING BOOK takes the reader from an initial understanding of the reality of elder abuse, through a discipline-specific treatise by an attorney, a physician, a nurse, and a social worker, to their final critical and reflective discussion on the benefits of multidisciplinary teams. Timely and insightful, this book is ESSEN-TIAL READING FOR CLINICIANS, EDUCATORS, RESEARCHERS, COMMUNITY AGENCIES, STUDENTS, and indeed, anyone concerned about older people and keeping them out of harm's way."

Elizabeth Podnieks, RN, EdD
Professor,
Ryerson University,
School of Nursing

The Haworth Press, Inc.
New York

The Clinical Management of Elder Abuse

The Clinical Management of Elder Abuse has been co-published simultaneously as *Clinical Gerontologist*, Volume 28, Numbers 1/2 2005.

The *Clinical Gerontologist* Monographic "Separates"

Below is a list of "separates," which in serials librarianship means a special issue simultaneously published as a special journal issue or double-issue and as a "separate" hardbound monograph. (This is a format which we also call a "DocuSerial.")

"Separates" are published because specialized libraries or professionals may wish to purchase a specific thematic issue by itself in a format which can be separately cataloged and shelved, as opposed to purchasing the journal on an on-going basis. Faculty members may also more easily consider a "separate" for classroom adoption.

"Separates" are carefully classified separately with the major book jobbers so that the journal tie-in can be noted on new book order slips to avoid duplicate purchasing.

You may wish to visit Haworth's website at . . .

http://www.HaworthPress.com

. . . to search our online catalog for complete tables of contents of these separates and related publications.

You may also call 1-800-HAWORTH (outside US/Canada: 607-722-5857), or Fax 1-800-895-0582 (outside US/Canada: 607-771-0012), or E-mail at:

docdelivery@haworthpress.com

The Clinical Management of Elder Abuse, edited by Georgia J. Anetzberger, PhD, ACSW, LISW (Vol. 28, No. 1/2, 2005). *As the baby boom generation ages, incidents of elder abuse are certain to continue to increase. Whether you are a student, an educator, an experienced clinician, or a novice in the field,* The Clinical Management of Elder Abuse *is a resource that you'll return to again and again as you work to improve the lives of this important growing population.*

Emerging Trends in Psychological Practice in Long-Term Care, edited by Margaret P. Norris, PhD, Victor Molinari, PhD, and Suzann M. Ogland-Hand, PhD (Vol. 25, No. 1/2/3/4, 2002). *"THEORY AND PRACTICAL APPLICATION ARE WELL BALANCED IN THIS BOOK, with case examples translating ideas into direct clinical implementation." (Nicholas C. Stilwell, PhD, Vice President, Psychology Associates of Bethlehem P.C.; Affiliate Staff Psychologist, St. Luke's Hospital, Bethlehem, Pennsylvania)*

Holocaust Survivors' Mental Health, edited by T. L. Brink, PhD (Vol. 14, No. 3, 1994). *"More than just another work about the Holocaust or post-traumatic stress disorder, this volume represents a scholarly effort to continue the ongoing and necessary research concerning the mental health of Holocaust survivors. . . . One of the most valuable parts of this book is the appendix of both Yiddish and Hebrew versions of mental status examinations and a depressive scale." (Journal of the American Medical Association)*

The Forgotten Aged: Ethnic, Psychiatric, and Societal Minorities, edited by T. L. Brink, PhD (Vol. 14, No. 1, 1994). *"A gripping 'read' giving glimpses of the less-known, old-age realities that are poignant, sad, but at times uplifting. . . . Should interest social workers and psychogeriatricians and should also be read by geriatricians who frequently encounter the dilemmas sensitively discussed in this book." (Age and Ageing)*

Hispanic Aged Mental Health, edited by T. L. Brink, PhD (Vol. 11, No. 3/4, 1992). *"Whether one is a research investigator or a practicing therapist, the specific information is useful and pertinent. Utilizing the information included in this text will greatly enhance working with this population of older patients whatever the ethnic and cultural background of the reader. Dr. Brink has done an outstanding job in producing a key reference in the field." (International Psychogeriatrics)*

Mental Health in the Nursing Home, edited by T. L. Brink, PhD (Vol. 9, No. 3/4, 1990). *"Modern in content and stimulating toward the innovation of nursing homes which escape becoming administratively stale institutions which simply warehouse their physically and mentally impaired population. It is the kind of book that prods inactive administrators to activate the steward's desk and go on into self-satisfying and patient-satisfying progress–both with and beyond experimentation." (Journal of the American Association of Psychiatric Administration)*

The Elderly Uncooperative Patient, edited by T. L. Brink, PhD (Vol. 6, No. 2, 1987). *"Contains down-to-earth, practical recommendations . . . recommended not only for administrators, but all personnel involved in the management of such patients." (Journal of the American Association of Psychiatric Administrators)*

Clinical Gerontology: A Guide to Assessment and Intervention, edited by T. L. Brink, PhD (Vol. 5, No. 1/2/3/4, 1986). *"A diverse array of important and useful information for practicing clinicians in the field of psychogeriatrics. The section on depression scales for use in later life is one of the best that I have read, covering several old and new assessment methods which could be used in practice as well as research. The book is useful for psychologists who are working with old people and will find a place as a textbook in postgraduate courses." (Australian Psychologist)*

The Clinical Management
of Elder Abuse

Georgia J. Anetzberger, PhD, ACSW, LISW
Editor

The Clinical Management of Elder Abuse has been co-published simultaneously as *Clinical Gerontologist*, Volume 28, Numbers 1/2 2005.

The Haworth Press, Inc.

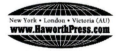

New York • London • Victoria (AU)
www.HaworthPress.com

The Clinical Management of Elder Abuse has been co-published simultaneously as *Clinical Gerontologist*™, Volume 28, Numbers 1/2 2005.

The Haworth Press, Inc., 10 Alice Street, Binghamton, NY 13904-1580 USA

Cover design by Jennifer Gaska

Library of Congress Cataloging-in-Publication Data

The clinical management of elder abuse / Georgia J. Anetzberger, editor.
     p. ; cm.–(Clinical gerontologist; v. 28, no. 1/2)
    Includes bibliographical references and index.
    ISBN 0-7890-1946-9 (hard cover : alk. paper)–ISBN 0-7890-1947-7 (soft cover : alk. paper)
    1. Aged–Abuse of. 2. Abused aged–Services for.
    [DNLM: 1. Elder Abuse–prevention & control–United States. 2. Elder Abuse–legislation & jurisprudence–United States. WT 30 C6413 2003] I. Anetzberger, Georgia J. (Georgia Jean) II. Series.
HV6626.3.C558 2003
362. 6–dc22
                                       2003016304

Indexing, Abstracting & Website/Internet Coverage

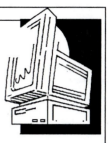

Clinical Gerontologist

This section provides you with a list of major indexing & abstracting services. That is to say, each service began covering this periodical during the year noted in the right column. Most Websites which are listed below have indicated that they will either post, disseminate, compile, archive, cite or alert their own Website users with research-based content from this work. (This list is as current as the copyright date of this publication.)

Abstracting, Website/Indexing Coverage . . . . Year When Coverage Began

- *Abstracts in Social Gerontology: Current Literature on Aging* 1989
- *Academic Abstracts/CD-ROM* 1995
- *Adis International Ltd* 1998
- *AgeInfo CD-ROM* 1995
- *AgeLine Database* 1982
- *AIDS and Cancer Research <http://www.csa.com>* 2003
- *Alzheimer's Disease Education & Referral Center (ADEAR)* 1995
- *Applied Social Sciences Index & Abstracts (ASSIA) (Online: ASSI via Data-Star) (CDRom: ASSIA Plus) <http://www.csa.com>* 1993
- *Behavioral Medicine Abstracts* 1982
- *CINAHL (Cumulative Index to Nursing & Allied Health Literature), in print, EBSCO, and SilverPlatter, Data-Star, and PaperChase.(Support materials include Subject Heading List,Database Search Guide, and instructional video.) <http://www.cinahl.com>* 1991
- *CNPIEC Reference Guide: Chinese National Directory of Foreign Periodicals* 1995
- *EMBASE/Excerpta Medica Secondary Publishing Division < http://www.elsevier.nl>* 1982
- *Environmental Sciences and Pollution Management (Cambridge Scientific Abstracts Internet Database Service) <http://www.csa.com>* 2003

(continued)

(continued)

*Exact start date to come.

Special Bibliographic Notes related to special journal issues
(separates) and indexing/abstracting:

- indexing/abstracting services in this list will also cover material in any "separate" that is co-published simultaneously with Haworth's special thematic journal issue or DocuSerial. Indexing/abstracting usually covers material at the article/chapter level.
- monographic co-editions are intended for either non-subscribers or libraries which intend to purchase a second copy for their circulating collections.
- monographic co-editions are reported to all jobbers/wholesalers/approval plans. The source journal is listed as the "series" to assist the prevention of duplicate purchasing in the same manner utilized for books-in-series.
- to facilitate user/access services all indexing/abstracting services are encouraged to utilize the co-indexing entry note indicated at the bottom of the first page of each article/chapter/contribution.
- this is intended to assist a library user of any reference tool (whether print, electronic, online, or CD-ROM) to locate the monographic version if the library has purchased this version but not a subscription to the source journal.
- individual articles/chapters in any Haworth publication are also available through the Haworth Document Delivery Services (HDDS).

The Clinical Management of Elder Abuse

CONTENTS

ABOUT THE EDITOR

Georgia J. Anetzberger, PhD, ACSW, LISW, is a consultant in private practice, a Research Associate with the Visiting Nurse Association Healthcare Partners of Ohio, an Adjunct Assistant Professor of Medicine at Case Western Reserve University, a member of the University Graduate Faculty in Health Care Administration at Cleveland State University, and a Fellow in the Gerontological Society of America. She has spent over 25 years addressing the problem of elder abuse, initially as an adult protective services worker and most recently as a researcher, administrator, and educator concerned with the dynamics of elder abuse situations. She has authored more than 30 publications on elder abuse or related interventions. Her work has appeared in *The Gerontologist, Violence Against Women, Generations,* and the *Journal of Cross-Cultural Gerontology.* A long-time Consulting Editor for the *Journal of Elder Abuse & Neglect,* she currently serves as the journal's Interim Co-Editor.

Dr. Anetzberger was the architect of Ohio's protective services law for adults and established the Ohio Coalition for Adult Protective Services and Consortium Against Adult Abuse (both affiliates of the National Committee for the Prevention of Elder Abuse, of which she is an officer). She has served on various national and state forums concerned with elder abuse, including research panels for the National Institute on Aging and the National Aging Resource Center on Elder Abuse as well as policy panels of the National Policy Summit on Elder Abuse and the Ohio Governor's Task Force on Family Violence. Dr. Anetzberger has presented on the topics of elder abuse and adult protective services for various local or national groups, including the American Society on Aging, the Gerontological Society of America, the American Counseling Association, and the National Association of Area Agencies on Aging.

Preface

Every day thousands of older Americans experience elder abuse. Some are beaten; others are denied life necessities. Some are abandoned; others are threatened or demeaned. Some are sexually assaulted; still others have their money or possessions taken from them. Their demographics and backgrounds may differ, but elder abuse victims share the serious consequences of the acts perpetrated against them, usually by family members or caregivers. They also share in the need for help that can treat the problem and prevent its recurrence.

Fortunately most elder abuse victims have contact with someone who can help, often clinicians in health and social services. These individuals have professional roles and legal responsibility in the clinical management of elder abuse situations. They are found in various practice settings and represent numerous disciplines. This publication is for them.

The intent of *The Clinical Management of Elder Abuse* is to provide professionals in clinical practice who work with older people an understanding of elder abuse and strategies for addressing the problem. The publication begins with a portrayal of elder abuse, first as evidenced through research and second as experienced by clinicians and victims. It considers clinical management of elder abuse in five steps that are described with regard to purpose, issues, and approaches: detection, assessment, planning, intervention, and follow-up. Three case studies are offered, which reflect various elder abuse forms and dynamics. They are clinically analyzed by helping professions likely to have contact with elder abuse victims: law, medicine, nursing, and social work. Initially this is accomplished by each clinician author providing a discipline-specific perspective on the case studies. Later the concept of multidisciplinary teams (M-teams) for elder abuse clinical management is introduced. The same clinicians are assembled and their comments recorded for collective analysis of the three case studies.

[Haworth co-indexing entry note]: "Preface." Anetzberger, Georgia J. Co-published simultaneously in *Clinical Gerontologist* (The Haworth Press, Inc.) Vol. 28, No. 1/2, 2005, pp. xv-xvi; and: *The Clinical Management of Elder Abuse* (ed: Georgia J. Anetzberger) The Haworth Press, Inc., 2005, pp. xiii-xiv. Single or multiple copies of this article are available for a fee from The Haworth Document Delivery Service [1-800-HAWORTH, 9:00 a.m. - 5:00 p.m. (EST). E-mail address: docdelivery@haworthpress.com].

http://www.haworthpress.com/web/CG   *xiii*

All of the contributors to *The Clinical Management of Elder Abuse* are or have been both clinicians and educators. Therefore, this publication represents our personal commitment to improving elder abuse practice by educating colleagues who struggle with these difficult situations in the regular course of their work. That said, we agree that nothing magical can be or is offered for quick or easy problem resolution. Rather, the publication's contents contain suggestions, techniques, and frameworks for making decisions and taking action. Together they provide a starting point upon which clinicians can build, using their own experiences and accumulated wisdom.

As Editor for *The Clinical Management of Elder Abuse*, I want to thank Maria Schimer, John McGreevey, Carol Miller, and Carol Dayton for serving as contributing authors. It has been my privilege to know and collaborate with each for at least fifteen years. My respect for them as clinicians, and human beings, grows with every contact.

Finally, no publication happens without the help and support of the people with whom we live and work. Therefore, on behalf of the contributing authors and myself, this publication is dedicated to those whose names may not be ascribed to any particular article, but whose encouragement and contribution made it possible.

Georgia J. Anetzberger, PhD, ACSW, LISW

The Reality of Elder Abuse

Georgia J. Anetzberger, PhD, ACSW, LISW

SUMMARY. There are two primary sources for understanding the reality of elder abuse. The first is empirical and derived from scientific study of its nature and scope. The second is experiential and illustrated in the perspectives of clinicians who detect and treat it along with victims who suffer its infliction and consequences. Both sources of understanding are evidenced in this overview of elder abuse as a health and social problem for older Americans. In addition, the article outlines the history in recognizing elder abuse as a problem and in developing strategies to address it. *[Article copies available for a fee from The Haworth Document Delivery Service: 1-800-HAWORTH. E-mail address: <docdelivery@haworthpress.com> Website: <http://www.HaworthPress.com> © 2005 by The Haworth Press, Inc. All rights reserved.]*

KEYWORDS. Elder abuse, definition and forms, prevalence and incidence, risk factors, victim perspectives

UNDERSTANDING ELDER ABUSE

Elder abuse "came of age" as a recognized health and social problem during the 1980s. However, its antecedents are found in two earlier periods, the first dating as far back as the mid-twentieth century.

Georgia J. Anetzberger is Research Associate, Visiting Nurse Association, Healthcare Partners of Ohio, Cleveland, Ohio.

[Haworth co-indexing entry note]: "The Reality of Elder Abuse." Anetzberger, Georgia J. Co-published simultaneously in *Clinical Gerontologist* (The Haworth Press, Inc.) Vol. 28, No. 1/2, 2005, pp. 1-25; and: *The Clinical Management of Elder Abuse* (ed: Georgia J. Anetzberger) The Haworth Press, Inc., 2005, pp. 1-25. Single or multiple copies of this article are available for a fee from The Haworth Document Delivery Service [1-800-HAWORTH, 9:00 a.m. - 5:00 p.m. (EST). E-mail address: docdelivery@haworthpress.com].

http://www.haworthpress.com/web/CG
Digital Object Identifier: 10.1300/J018v28n01_01

The expansion of public benefits in the 1950s enabled more older people to live on their own in the community. Professionals across service sectors, from banking and insurance to social work and law, became especially concerned about the growing number of mentally impaired older people living alone, often without nearby family support. It was feared that many could not provide for their own care or protection without community intervention (American Public Welfare Association, 1962; O'Neill, 1965). Dialogues at local and national levels on the need for protective services to address the potential neglect and exploitation of these vulnerable adults led to demonstration projects aimed at delineating the intervention and its clientele as well as evaluating its effectiveness (Horowitz & Estes, 1971; Blenkner et al., 1974; US Senate Special Committee on Aging, 1977). From this inception, adult protective services spread across the country during the mid-1970s, largely as a public agency responsibility, fueled by federal funding through Title XX of the Social Security Act (since 1981 incorporated into the Social Services Block Grant) (Brody, 1977; Regan, 1978).

The second antecedent period in recognizing elder abuse as a problem for older people sprang out of medicine, with four 1975 publications. Butler (1975) expressed alarm about "a battered old person syndrome" in his Pulitzer Prize-winning book *Why Survive? Being Old in America*; Clark, Mankikar, and Gray (1975) discovered a "Diogenes syndrome" wherein unkempt older people live in filth and debris and show no shame for their situation; and Baker (1975) and Burston (1975) in Great Britain labeled family members who physically abuse elderly relatives "granny batterers." Research on a broadening concept of elder abuse began shortly thereafter, with only a handful of studies completed by 1980 (Lau & Kosberg, 1979; Block & Sinnott, 1979; O'Malley et al., 1979; Douglass, Hickey, & Noel, 1980). These investigations were limited methodologically and focused primarily on exploring the forms of elder abuse and the characteristics of victims and perpetrators. Nonetheless, they were sufficient to trigger Congressional hearings on the subject along with increasing media coverage and presentations at professional associations (US House Select Committee on Aging and US House Science and Technology Subcommittee, 1978; US House Select Committee on Aging, 1980).

The 1980s are widely acknowledged as the decade for public awakening and broadening professional action regarding elder abuse (Wolf, 1988; Roybal, 1991). Certainly by the end of that decade elder abuse was recognized as a major issue of older Americans and an important aspect of family violence. Many of the key elder abuse studies were published during the 1980s which shape our understanding of this phenomenon even today (e.g., Sengstock & Liang, 1982; Phillips, 1988; Wolf, Godkin, & Pillemer, 1984; Anetzberger, 1987; Pillemer & Finkelhor, 1988; Steinmetz, 1988). Several federal policies for addressing the problem were enacted, including provisions around elder abuse prevention, in Older Americans Act reauthorization and identification of older people as a potential targeted group for funding, in Family Violence Prevention and Services Act amendment. The majority of states and United States territories passed adult protective services or elder abuse reporting laws (Tatara, 1995). Finally, Haworth Press launched the *Journal of Elder Abuse & Neglect*, the Clearinghouse on Abuse and Neglect of the Elderly (CANE) was underway at the University of Delaware, the National Center for the Prevention of Elder Abuse was established, many state or local elder abuse coalitions were created, and numerous training or demonstration projects on elder abuse prevention or treatment were publicly funded (Wolf & Nerenberg, 1994).

Since the 1980s the field of elder abuse has sprung tentacles, reaching across systems, settings, and continents. For example, the growing criminalization of elder abuse has expanded the networks of involved practitioners to include those in law enforcement and domestic violence programs. With them has come particular interest in areas of financial abuse like telemarketing fraud, sexual assault in late life, and battered older women (Wilber & Reynolds, 1996; Tueth, 2000; Ramsey-Klawsnik, 1991; Simmelink, 1996; Harris, 1996; Brandl & Raymond, 1997). In addition, although awareness of elder abuse in nursing homes and other institutional settings began in the 1970s with exposes of deplorable conditions (Townsend, 1971; Stannard, 1973; Mendelson, 1974), it has heightened in recent years as a result of investigations by Long Term Care Ombudsman Programs and Medical Fraud Abuse Units (Huber, Netting, & Kautz, 1996; Payne & Cikovic, 1995). Likewise, research on elder abuse in such other countries as Canada, Finland, Israel, India, and Japan reveals that the problem is global (Podnieks, 1992; Kivela et al., 1992; Kosberg & Garcia, 1995), and an international perspective and response is required (United Nations Economic and Social Council, 2002).

Definitions and Forms

There is no universally accepted definitions or set of forms for elder abuse. Many different ones have been used by researchers studying the problem and policymakers enacting related laws. The result is a general lack of comparability of research findings or state reporting statistics as well as confusion among practitioners and the public trying to understand elder abuse (Gelles & Cornell, 1985; Hudson, 1986; Wolf, 1988; Schene & Ward, 1988; Hudson, 1991).

Several controversies underlie the absence of universally accepted elder abuse definitions and forms. They include the following: How broad in meaning is elder abuse? Must there be intent for an act to be considered elder abuse? Does elder abuse always require a perpetrator? Who decides whether or not an act constitutes elder abuse? What is the onset age for elder abuse to occur? Should vulnerability of the victim be required in defining elder abuse? Do the effects, frequency, severity, or duration of the elder abuse play a role in defining the problem?

Some definitions of elder abuse limit themselves to a few select forms, and others include a wide range of forms. All elder abuse definitions used in research include physical abuse, and most also include neglect, psychological abuse, and financial abuse. Some research definitions incorporate sexual assault under physical abuse, and abandonment under neglect. Other times, these forms are investigated separately. Likewise, some research definitions separate neglect into two types, such as physical neglect and psychological neglect, or use the broader concept of exploitation and distinguish types within it, like financial abuse and violation of rights. Finally, many forms of elder abuse go by more than one name in the research literature. Psychological abuse, for instance, is sometimes referenced as emotional abuse or verbal abuse.

Like research definitions, definitions found in state elder abuse laws are most likely to include physical abuse, neglect, and financial abuse or exploitation as recognized forms. In fact, these forms are found in over three-fourths of the nation's 69 elder abuse laws (Tatara, 1995). Precise definitions are unique to each state. For example, Ohio's protective services law for adults (Ohio Revised Code 5105.60) contains definitions for abuse, exploitation, and neglect, i.e.,

- abuse: the infliction upon an adult by himself or others of injury, unreasonable confinement, intimidation, or cruel punishment with resulting physical harm, pain, or mental anguish.
- exploitation: the unlawful or improper act of a caretaker using an adult or his resources for monetary or personal benefit, profit, or gain.
- neglect: the failure of an adult to provide for himself the goods or services necessary to avoid physical harm, mental anguish, or mental illness or the failure of a caretaker to provide such goods or services.

Although not expressly listed, Ohio's definition of abuse encompasses self-abuse, physical abuse, psychological abuse, and sexual assault. Exploitation addresses both financial abuse and violation of rights, and neglect includes self-neglect, physical neglect, psychological neglect, and some instances of abandonment. Moreover, acts of elder abuse must have consequences in order for them to come under the purview of Ohio law.

Federal policy on elder abuse is evident in the Older Americans Act, which includes definitions of the problem in the 1987 amendments. The Act recognizes physical abuse, neglect, and exploitation. However, the definitions of these forms are sufficiently broad to contain self-abuse, self-neglect, psychological abuse, and physical neglect as well.

No forms of elder abuse are more controversial than self-abuse and self-neglect. Some researchers and policymakers believe that the act of elder abuse requires a perpetrator, and the perpetrator must be someone other than the recipient of the elder abuse her/himself. They, therefore, exclude self-abuse and self-neglect from definitions of elder abuse, often considering them issues of inadequate care or support, which require different approaches for intervention than other elder abuse forms (Fulmer & O'Malley, 1987; Johnson, 1991). Still, 40 states have elder abuse laws that cover self-neglect, and Montana mandates the provision of services to self-neglecting older people, although it has no elder abuse law covering self-neglect (Tatara, 1995).

Since the mid-1980s research and public policy forums on elder abuse have recommended the adoption of elder abuse definitions that are clear, uniform, and relevant to practice (University of New Hampshire; 1986; Stein, 1991; US Department of Health and Human Services, 1992; Watson, 1995; National Research Council, 2003). Johnson (1986) and Hudson (1991) are recognized for their pioneering attempts to standardize elder abuse definitions through research. Hudson, for instance, conducted a three-round Delphi survey with a national panel of elder abuse experts to develop a taxonomy of elder abuse and definitions of related concepts. The result was a five-level taxonomy and eleven definitions. In the taxonomy Level I concerns violence involving older persons, Level II considers the relationship between victim and perpetrator, Level III relates to how the destructive behavior is carried out, Level IV surrounds the purpose motivating this destructive behavior, and Level V identifies the specific type of destructive behavior. Much of Hudson's subsequent research has expanded upon this study, comparing the perception of these national elder abuse experts in defining the problem to public perceptions across ages and cultures (Hudson et al., 1998, 2000; Hudson & Carlson, 1999).

Widely accepted organizationally-based definitions also exist. For example, after analyzing federal and state elder abuse definitions in law, the National Center on Elder Abuse (1999) identified specific definitions for physical abuse, sexual abuse, emotional abuse, financial/material exploitation, neglect, abandonment, and self-neglect. At the state level, an Ohio team of researchers, operating under a statewide roundtable convened by the Ohio Department of Human Services (now called the Ohio Department of Job and Family Services), identified definitions for elder abuse and ten distinct forms. This occurred in the process of developing and testing screening tools and a referral protocol for service providers that involved practitioner key informant interviews, focus groups, and product application. The definitions are found in Figure 1 (Anetzberger et al., 1999; Anetzberger, 2001; Bass et al., 2001). These definitions for elder abuse, along with the specific definitions for abuse, neglect, and exploitation contained in Ohio law, will provide the framework for clinical analysis and management in the set of articles to follow.

Prevalence and Incidence

Because there has never been a national study on the prevalence of elder abuse in the United States, prevalence statistics offered for the problem tend to be based upon localized research. Collectively these studies suggest a prevalence rate between one and ten percent of the older people surveyed or older Americans as a whole (Lau & Kosberg, 1979; Block & Sinnett, 1979; McLaughlin, Nickell, & Gill, 1980; Gioglio & Blakemore, 1983; Pillemer & Finkelhor, 1988). Pillemer and Finkelhor (1988) conducted the best known and best regarded of the localized prevalence studies, surveying 2,020 randomly selected community-dwelling older persons in the metropolitan Boston area. Respondents were asked about three elder abuse forms: physical abuse, chronic verbal aggression, and neglect. Among the subjects, 3.2 percent experienced at least one form since age 65, with physical abuse (2.2 percent) more common than either verbal aggression (1.1 percent) or neglect (0.4 percent). Using somewhat similar methodologies but typically including financial abuse among the forms investigated, prevalence rates for elder abuse of between four and six percent were found in Canada, Great Britain, Finland, and the Netherlands (Podnieks, 1992; Ogg & Bennett, 1992; Kivela et al., 1992; Comijs et al., 1998). Financial abuse or verbal aggression tended to be more common than the other elder abuse forms in these studies.

FIGURE 1. Elder Abuse Forms and Definitions

Elder Abuse

- The infliction of injury or suffering on a person age 60 years or older by her/himself or another person.

Physical Abuse

- Abuse by others: Infliction of injury or pain on an older person by another person.
- Self-abuse: A form of physical abuse that occurs when an older person inflicts injury or pain on her/himself.
- Sexual abuse: Contact of a sexual nature that is forced, uninvited, or administered unknowingly through deception.

Psychological Abuse

- Infliction of mental anguish, use of threats, emotional abuse, forced witnessing of the abuse of others, isolation, or attacks against property and other acts of intimidation upon an older person by another person.

Neglect

- Physical neglect: Failure of a caregiver to provide an older person with necessary goods or services.
- Emotional neglect: Failure of a caregiver to provide adequate social or emotional support or stimulation to an older person.
- Abandonment: Desertion of an older person by a caregiver.
- Self-neglect: Failure of an older person to provide her/himself with necessary goods or services.

Exploitation

- Financial abuse: Unlawful or improper use of an older person's property or resources.
- Violation of rights: Denying an older person rights conferred on her/him by law or legal process.

After reviewing references in the Library of Congress, surveying state human services departments, and holding hearings on the problem, the US House Select Committee on Aging (1990) estimated that five percent of older Americans may be victims of moderate to severe elder abuse, resulting in around 1.5 million victims annually. Several years later the National Center on Elder Abuse (1997) projected 2.16 million elder abuse victims, with self-neglect included. The Center's figures considered both research and state reporting data.

The National Center of Elder Abuse (1998) also completed the first national incidence study on elder abuse, investigating the number of unduplicated new cases of domestic elder abuse among persons age 60 and above in 1996. In conducting the research, it used a representative sample of 20 counties in 15 states and considered two data sources: reports to adult protective services and reports from sentinels (i.e., specifically trained individuals in community agencies having frequent contact with older people). The results of this study suggested a 1996 national elder abuse incidence rate of 551,011. Only 21 percent of the total were reported to and subsequently substantiated by adult protective services agencies. Of these, 38.4 percent represented self-neglect, 30.0 percent neglect, 21.8 percent emotional/psychological abuse, 18.6 percent financial/material exploitation, and 15.8 percent physical abuse.

As evident from the National Elder Abuse Incidence Study, most elder abuse is not reported to authorities charged with its investigation, like adult protective services. The US House Select Committee on Aging (1990) estimates that only one in eight cases are reported. However, based upon their Boston prevalence data, Pillemer and Finkelhor (1988) suggest that actual reporting may be even lower; perhaps only one in 14 elder abuse situations are ever reported to authorities.

Since the mid-1980s reports of domestic elder abuse to state adult protective services or aging agencies have steadily increased (Teaster, 2003). Nationwide 293,000 reports were received in 1996, compared to 117,000 in 1986, a 150.4 percent increase over a decade. Nearly two-thirds of reports were substantiated. One third of these cases were self-neglect or self-abuse, by far the most commonly reported forms of elder abuse and growing among reports received. From 1990 to 1996 reports of neglect (including self-neglect) increased while those of physical abuse, exploitation, and emotional abuse decreased. Reports of sexual abuse remained constant at 0.3 percent of total reports over this period (Tatara & Kuzmeskus, 1997; Tatara, 1996).

Reporting trends vary by state, with some states noticing declines in recent years. For instance, Ohio adult protective services agencies received 15,505 elder abuse reports in state fiscal year 1996, but only 12,194 in 2000, a decrease of over 25 percent. Among any ten elder abuse reports in Ohio, six tend to concern self-neglect, two surround neglect by a caregiver, and one each address abuse and exploitation. Within the period 1996-2000 reports of self-neglect increased, while those of abuse, neglect, and exploitation decreased (Ohio Department of Human Services, 1996; Ohio Department of Job and Family Services, 2000).

Reports of elder abuse come primarily from health and social services providers, especially those who offer care in the homes of older persons. Some practitioners, like visiting nurses and social work case managers, are more likely to report than others, such as attorneys, members of the clergy, or physicians (Dolon & Hendricks, 1989; Blakely & Dolon, 1991; Rosenblatt, Cho, & Durance, 1996; National Center on Elder Abuse, 1997; Teaster, 2003).

There are many reasons why practitioners fail to report elder abuse, despite the fact that nearly all states mandate reporting by professionals (Tatara, 1995). These reasons include the following: lack of awareness about reporting responsibilities or elder abuse as a problem, perception that reporting abridges client confidentiality or destroys established rapport with the client, fear of litigation or other reprisal by the victim or perpetrator, lack of faith in the agency charged with handling the report or those providing services to protect the victim, or belief that reporting runs counter to such personal values as sanctity of the family (Gilbert, 1986; Fulmer & O'Malley, 1987; Thobaben, 1989; Daniels, Baumhover, & Clark-Daniels, 1989; Anetzberger, 1992; Coyne, Petenza, & Berbig, 1996).

Elder abuse laws with mandatory reporting provisions were enacted to foster professional case finding and referral to agencies responsible for assisting victims (Zborowsky, 1985; Regan, 1990). Various studies, however, suggest that mandatory reporting increases neither professional reporting nor the rate of elder abuse substantiation; rather, professional and public awareness is seen as key to case identification (Wolf, Godkin, & Pillemer, 1986; Fredriksen, 1989; US General Accounting Office, 1991).

Mandatory reporting provisions have been subject to controversy since they were first contained in elder abuse laws (Faulkner, 1982; Kapp, 1995). The controversy surrounding them includes the following: vague definitions for elder abuse identification, potential for inappropriately labeling persons as perpetrators, lack of adequate funding for proper law implementation, and undermining the autonomy of older people (Callahan, 1988; Blanton, 1989; Daniels, Baumhover, & Clark-Daniels, 1989; Macolini, 1995).

Elder Abuse Diagnosis and Risk Factors

Several theoretical perspectives have been suggested for understanding elder abuse (see Figure 2) (Phillips, 1986; Gelles, 1991; Nadien, 1995; Ansello, 1996; Aitken & Griffin, 1996; Wieche, 1998; Carp, 2000). Some are borrowed from the family violence literature explaining abuse against other populations, particularly children. Some have received support from empirical study, like psychopathology theory (Wolf, Godkin, & Pillemer, 1984; Anetzberger, 1987) and symbolic interactionism

(Steinmetz, 1988). Some have been collapsed into operational formulas for elder abuse interventions, such as situational, vulnerability, and exchange theories into the environmental press model (Ansello, 1996). However, none of the theoretical perspectives has been rigorously tested (National Research Council, 2003). In addition, with a problem as complex as elder abuse, it is unlikely that any single theoretical perspective could explain all forms and situations.

Lacking an established theoretical base for explaining elder abuse, research has focused on characterizing the victim and perpetrator, including identifying the risk factors which seem to increase the likelihood of abuse occurrence.

Summaries of research on elder abuse risk factors suggest that those related to the perpetrator are more predictive of abuse occurrence than those related to the victim. Johnson (1991) reviewed nine published works on elder abuse and ranked commonly identified characteristics for perpetrators and victims. There were at least four citations for each of the following perpetrator characteristics: psychopathology, stress/ burnout, financial dependence, and dependencies other than financial. There was less consensus about victim characteristics, with only two receiving at least three citations: impairment and dependence. Lachs and Pillemer (1995) identified eight salient risk factors from the elder abuse literature, but concluded that the three most important factors rest with the perpetrator: substance abuse or mental illness, perpetrator dependence on the victim, and history of violence or extrafamilial antisocial behavior. The other five salient risk factors follow: poor health and functional impairment of the victim, cognitive impairment of the victim, shared living arrangements, external factors causing stress, and social isolation. Finally, from research using a validated assessment instrument, Reis and Nahmiash (1998) identified several risk factors related to the perpetrator, but only two related to the victim. For perpetrators in a caregiving relationship with victims, perpetrator risk factors include: substance abuse, mental health disorders, and behavioral problems; poor interpersonal relations; mental or family conflict; inexperience or reluctance to perform the caregiving role; lack of empathy or understanding for the care recipient; and financial dependence on the victim. Risks factors related to the victim are past elder abuse and lack of social support.

Various conceptual frameworks have been developed for viewing victim and perpetrator characteristics. An early one developed by Rathbone-McCuan and Hashimi (1982) focused on isolators (biophysical, psychological, economic, and social) in the lives of elder abuse victims.

FIGURE 2. Theoretical Perspectives for Understanding Elder Abuse

Conflict theory: Given imbalances in scarce resources, the potential exists for someone to take advantage of an older person.

Ecology theory: Abuse results from disorientation when sudden, unwanted change makes existing rules of behavior no longer workable.

Exchange theory: Older people are dependent upon those who abuse them out of a sense of power or power loss, but find the cost in terms of the abuse is less than a benefit of receiving care.

Feminist theory: Abuse against women results from structural inequities in society that disadvantage women.

Functionalism: Abuse exists because of cultural norms that leave few choices outside of the family to provide care for elderly members.

Psychopathology theory: Problems in psychosocial functioning can promote or provoke elder abuse.

Role theory: Elder abuse results from the inadequate, inappropriate, or unwilling provision of care.

Situational theory: Circumstances, such as social isolation or excessive stress upon a caregiver, can render an older person vulnerable to abuse.

Social learning theory: Abuse is learned from and reinforced by those of perceived authority.

Symbolic interactionism: Abuse is situationally defined and occurs in social interactions when there exist discrepancies between behaviors and role expectations.

Vulnerability theory: Impairment and incapacity can render older people at risk of abuse.

Anetzberger (1990) considered vulnerability to elder abuse as resulting from characteristics of the individual (personal, situational, environmental, and cultural) or characteristics of the system (inadequate funding, inappropriate services, and premature policy and practice). Lastly, Kosberg and Nahmiash (1996) identified characteristics of victims, perpetrators, and the abuse milieu in their conceptual framework. Those for victims include: gender, mental status, health, age, substance abuse, living arrangements, psychological factors, problem behaviors, dependence, and isolation. Those for perpetrators include: substance abuse, mental or emotional illness, lack of caregiving experience, reluctance, history of abuse, stress and burden, dependency, dementia, personality traits, and lack of social support. Characteristics for the milieu of abuse surround either the social context (financial problems, family violence, lack of social support, family disharmony, and living arrangements) or cultural norms (ageism, sexism, attitudes toward violence, reactions to abuse, attitudes toward persons with disabilities, and family caregiving imperatives).

From research and reported cases a profile emerges of the typical elder abuse victim. In general that person is a woman age 75 or older who is widowed and living in her own home. She experiences more than one form of elder abuse, and has suffered multiple occurrences of the problem over time. Her perpetrator is a family member, usually either her adult child or spouse. That person also is typically male and living with the victim (e.g., Wolf, Godkin, & Pillemer, 1986; Tatara & Kuzmeskus, 1997; Lachs et al., 1997; National Center on Elder Abuse, 1998; Teaster, 2003).

There is recognition and some empirical evidence that risk factors and victim/perpetrator profiles vary by form of elder abuse (Steinmetz, 1988; Dolon & Blakely, 1989). For example, Wolf, Godkin, and Pillemer (1986) found differences in both for physical abuse, psychological abuse, material abuse, active neglect, and passive neglect in their research on three model elder abuse intervention projects. To illustrate, physical abuse victims tended to be younger, married, more independent in their functioning, in poor emotional health, and with stable social support. Their perpetrators had histories of mental illness or alcohol abuse, recent health decline, increased dependency, and poor relations with the victims. By contrast, victims of passive neglect tended to be older, unmarried, functionally impaired, and experiencing a loss of social supports. Their perpetrators lived with them, had unrealistic expectations, and had recent medical complaints. They also evidenced no financial dependency and had good relations with the victims. However, they found the victims to be sources of stress at a time they suffered from a loss of social support.

Anetzberger (2000) attempted to converge empirical data on both risk factors and victim/perpetrator characteristics to propose an explanatory model for elder abuse. The model has application to understanding elder abuse as it manifests itself across forms, settings, and relationships. It suggests that elder abuse is primarily a function of characteristics on the part of the perpetrator and secondarily on those of the victim. These merge and provide the underlying etiology for abuse occurrence. However, context is important as well, initially that which brings the victim and perpetrator together (such as spousal relations or adult children residing in the homes of elderly parents) and later that which triggers the occurrence of abuse (such as the repeated refusal of the victim to comply with caregiver expectations or the perpetrator being alone with easily accessible valuables).

However, beyond history and definitions, forms and statistics, theoretical perspectives and profiles are individual persons, each one experiencing elder abuse uniquely. The meaning of elder abuse for parties intimately involved in the problem is the focus of the sections which follow. Two perspectives are discussed: that of the clinician faced with elder abuse detection and intervention and that of the victim suffering its effects.

EXPERIENCING ELDER ABUSE

The Clinician's Perspective

Even to professional clinicians having experience in managing difficult client situations, elder abuse is perplexing, complex, and ethically charged. It can be hard to detect, with subtle manifestations or signs that mirror other problems or illnesses. It can seem impossible to control, particularly when the victim refuses help or denies the seriousness of mistreatment.

Elder abuse takes many different forms, and frequently does in any situation. It may involve more than one perpetrator and can continue or reoccur across time, and even across settings. Moreover, decision-making related to elder abuse interventions is rarely easy and is frequently clouded by ethical dilemmas. For example, deciding if and when to report an incident to authorities may be affected by numerous factors, including concern for possible repercussions against the victim or the effect of incorrectly labeling a perpetrator.

Beyond the dynamics of clinically managing elder abuse situations are the sensations and the emotions that they engender. Standing in a home inhabited by a self-neglecting elder person can be an assault upon the sense of smell. The stench of rotting garbage or flesh, animal defecation or urine-soaked mattresses, burnt furniture or moldy books can fill nasal cavities and remain in memory, and on clothing, long after the visit ends. Addressing caregiver neglect situations can leave clinicians emotionally spent–questioning how things deteriorated so badly, struggling to help victims understand their options, fearing the consequences of inaction, and wrestling with the concepts of autonomy versus safety in determining appropriate intervention.

Involvement in cases of physical abuse challenges the sense of sight. Open wounds, bruises at various stages of healing, and burnt skin may cover the color spectrum and make observers wince. They also can engulf clinicians with an urgency that "something must be done now" and anger when it isn't. Psychological abuse bombards the sense of hearing with messages at once so damning and so incredible that clinicians may feel vulnerable themselves encountering them. Words that discredit, demean, or threaten rob victims' souls, leaving them feeling worthless, depressed, or anxious. They also can make clinicians feel like moral police for interfering and conspirators for not. Finally, situations of financial abuse tax the mind, searching for clues and solving puzzles. Hidden by family ties or among stacks of unpaid bills, evidenced only in the occasional missing check or altered document, financial abuse requires intellect to unravel and sometimes cultural distance to recognize amidst the American values of materialism, status, and individual acquisition that often foster it.

Reactions to elder abuse among clinicians are far-ranging. Some are repulsed by such situations. They want nothing to do with them, occasionally blaming the victims as either bringing the problem on themselves or capable of resolving it, if they only tried. Other clinicians have filters–cultural, professional, or personal–which enable them to encounter elder abuse situations and somehow remain oblivious to their damaging, potentially lethal, consequences. Still others follow legal mandates or professional standards, educating themselves about elder abuse and reporting it when necessary, but electing to keep a distance. For them, the nature of the problem is too horrendous or consuming to allow it more than minimal entry into the psyche.

There are some clinicians, however, albeit fewer than are needed, for whom addressing elder abuse is a calling and a passion. Within the context of their chosen professions, they have committed themselves to understanding the problem and taking whatever measures are appropriate to identify, prevent, and treat it. Colleagues often fail to comprehend a calling or passion for a problem always challenging, and frequently disheartening. They recognize that there are no simple cures or easy wins with elder abuse. There are even fewer expressions of gratitude. Accusations of intrusiveness are more likely. These colleagues know that it can be frightening to be wrong in assessing elder abuse, but perhaps less so than being right. Furthermore, most situations require considerable time and skills typically not employed in customary care or service delivery.

For clinicians who have committed themselves to addressing elder abuse as a calling, there are rewards, although they may not be publicly recognized or acknowledged. Focusing on social workers who provide adult protective services, McLaughlin (1988:32) concludes:

Perhaps the most reported attribute of a skilled and effective protective service worker is taught in no university. It can't be found in any book or journal article. That attribute is courage. To successfully fulfill their responsibility to the victims of elder abuse, practitioners need the courage to allow competent clients to define for themselves what constitutes appropriate services. They need the courage to respect their client's wishes in the face of criticism from family members, the media, and powerful people in the community.

The difficulty of courageously managing elder abuse situations was recognized in the original development of adult protective services as a means to assist older people incapable of caring for themselves and lacking others able to provide support. In discussing the Benjamin Rose Institute's demonstration Protective Service Project, Wasser (1971: 521) noted "that the practitioner functions with a dual stream of opposing incentives, that of dealing with a protective client as a self-determining adult and, simultaneously, as one for whom serious interventions are required if he is to be helped to bring his disturbed and disturbing behavior under control." Unfortunately, serious interventions can be constrained by inadequate or inappropriate community resources or by unrealistic demands upon the time of the protective services workers (Anetzberger, 1990; Mixson, 1995). They also can be hampered by voluminous paperwork, personal and professional isolation, or role conflict, as protective services workers struggle between investigation/law enforcement and the provision of social services (Wynkoop & Gerstein, 1993; Otto, 2000).

The rewards for affording protection to elder abuse victims often tend to be intrinsic and reside in philosophical concepts of personal, societal, or religious importance, such as beneficence and justice (Johnson, 1999). They relate to a desire to "do good" or "make a difference," recognizing that the definition of these concepts varies by individual and situation. Furthermore, for those who chose the helping professions, reward also rests in risk reduction for vulnerable persons. The danger and extreme need of many elder abuse victims provide compelling justification for protective intervention. With the reduction or elimination of danger or need can come enormous personal satisfaction and sense of accomplishment for the clinician.

The Victim's Perspective

The meaning of elder abuse to victims has been captured in a variety of ways. Coverage by the mass media encompasses scenes of extreme neglect, including footage of sordid living conditions and courtroom proceedings against perpetrators, such as those presented by television's "20/20" on March 19, 1999 of the physical neglect and exploitation of former boxer Jimmy Bivens. Film portrayals include interviews with physical abuse victims, such as Terra Nova Film's seven-year chronology of Norman's physical abuse principally by his oldest son in "I'd Rather Be Home." Public testimonies cover the range of elder abuse forms and have been given during hearings conducted at every governmental level, including the US Congress from the 1970s onward.

Collectively these scenes, portrayals, and testimonies suggest that elder abuse situations are not the same. Each has its own origins and dynamics. Each impacts its victim distinctively, reflecting the uniqueness of that individual's background, personality, and circumstances. However, there are certain commonalities shared by victims that bear noting in any discussion on the reality of elder abuse. These commonalities are evidenced in the consequences or effects of elder abuse on victims. Furthermore, they are seen in the responses of victims to the infliction of abuse or neglect.

Anetzberger (1997) offers a conceptual framework for understanding the effects of elder abuse upon victims. It suggests that the meaning of abuse is influenced by the victim's cultural background, cohort grouping, and individual experiences. Meaning is modified by the nature of the abuse (including its type, severity, and duration), the victim's relationship with the perpetrator, and personal circumstances (such as social support network and disability status).

The importance of culture on the meaning and response to elder abuse has received increased attention in recent years (Stein, 1991; Archstone Foundation, 1998; Tatara, 1997, 1999). The findings of numerous studies across various cultural groups suggest that ethnic background, and such other cultural factors as sexual orientation and gender socialization, may result in differences in how victims define elder abuse and their help-seeking behavior (Brown, 1989; Griffin, 1994; Tomita, 1994; Nagpaul, 1997; Chang & Moon, 1997; Sanchez, 1999; Hudson & Carlson, 1999; Moon, Tomita & Jung-Kamei, 2001). For example, Moon and Williams (1993) found that Korean-American elders have a narrower definition of elder abuse and a greater reluctance to seek help than either Caucasian Americans or African-Americans. In addition, Cook-Daniels (1997) suggests that older gays and lesbians may be more vulnerable to elder abuse as a result of an unwillingness to seek assistance from social service providers after years of hiding and living in a homophobic environment. Even within ethnic or other cultural groups, meaning attached to elder abuse may vary by locale, history, or socioeconomic status (Krassen Maxwell & Maxwell, 1992; Hudson et al., 1998). For instance, Hudson and her associates (2000) observed within-group differences in the assessment of elder abuse vignettes among five Caucasian American groups in North Carolina.

Similarly, the collective values, attitudes, and experiences of a cohort or peer group can express themselves on the meaning and response victims give to elder abuse (Ramsey-Klawsnik, 1991; Anetzberger, Korbin, & Tomita, 1996). For example, today's elderly adults' connection with two World Wars and the Great Depression has resulted in an emphasis on social harmony, attachment to authority, and selfless contribution (Strauss & Howe, 1991), which may render them more willing to excuse violent behavior and remain in abuse situations if they believe that doing so promotes family stability or reflects religious doctrine.

The effects of elder abuse appear to assume four possible dimensions: physical, behavioral, psychological, and social (Lau & Kosberg, 1979; O'Malley et al., 1979; Sengstock & Liang, 1982; Pillemer, 1985; Hwalek, 1987; Quinn & Tomita, 1997; Anetzberger, 1997; Wolf, 1997). Besides injury or pain, physical effects include sleep disturbances, eating problems, and headaches. Behavioral effects include anger, helplessness, reduced coping, and suicidal actions. Psychological effects can be wide-ranging and include denial, fear, anxiety, and depression. Finally, social effects include dependence, withdrawal, and fewer contacts.

Little research has focused on the consequences of elder abuse (Wolf, 1997; National Research Council, 2003). Most evidence of its occurrence and typology comes from clinical records, case studies, or victim comment. Early investigations on elder abuse effects explored resulting depression (Phillips, 1983; Bristowe & Collins, 1989). For instance, in a comparison group study of elderly victims and nonvictims, Pillemer and Prescott (1989) found that victims of physical abuse, neglect, and chronic verbal aggression reported much higher levels of depression. Likewise, depression emerged as a consequence of marital violence among an elderly subsample from the National Family Violence Resurvey data (Harris, 1996). Netherlands research comparing elder abuse victims and non-victims showed more psychological distress among victims, with social support emerging as a favorable moderator (Comijs et al., 1999). In addition, Osgood and Manetta (2000-2001) studied older women who had been patients in psychiatric facilities and discovered that those who had thought about or attempted suicide were more likely to have been victimized by battery, rape, or child abuse. However, the consequences of abuse for older adults may be less than it is for younger adults. In comparing older and younger female trauma victims, Acierno and his associates (2002) found a lower incidence of depression and posttraumatic psychopathology among older victims.

Focusing on the physical effects of elder abuse, it is estimated that nearly 50 percent of all incidents result in physically apparent trauma (Floyd, 1984; Jones, 1988). As seen in hospital emergency departments, the most common manifestations of neglect are dehydration and malnutrition, and the most common physical injuries are bruises, lacerations, head injury, and fractures (Jones, 1990).

Victim response to elder abuse can range from denial or concealment to leaving the abusive situation or contacting authorities charged with investigating the problem. Research on victim response is as minimal as that on elder abuse effects. However, agency statistics and antidotal evidence suggest that few victims personally seek help for themselves from adult protective services, and fewer still elect emergency shelter through domestic violence programs (Salend et al., 1984; Nerenberg, 1996; National Center on Elder Abuse, 1998; Grossman & Lundy, 2003). Some studies indicate that older adults of Asian or Hispanic backgrounds prefer turning to family or friends for assistance, while African-Americans turn to others, such as formal service providers or the police (Moon & Williams, 1993; Anetzberger, Korbin, & Tomita, 1996).

REFERENCES

Acierno, R., Brady, K., Gray, M., Kilpatrick, D.G., Resnick, H., & Best, C.L. (2002). Psychopathology following interpersonal violence: A comparison of risk factors in older and younger adults. *Journal of Clinical Geropsychology, 8* (1), 13-23.

Aitken, L., & Griffin, G. (1996). *Gender issues in elder abuse.* London: Sage.

American Public Welfare Association. (1962). *Guide statement on protective services for older adults.* Chicago: Author.

Anetzberger, G.J. (1987). *The etiology of elder abuse by adult offspring.* Springfield, IL: Charles C Thomas.

Anetzberger, G.J. (1990). Abuse, neglect, and self-neglect: Issues of vulnerability. In Z. Harel, P. Ehrlich, & R. Hubbard (Eds.), *The vulnerable aged: People, services, and policies* (pp. 140-148). New York: Springer Publishing Company.

Anetzberger, G.J. (1992). *Elder abuse programming among Geriatric Education Centers: Final report to the Geriatric Initiatives Branch of the Bureau of Health Professions, US Department of Health and Human Services.* Cleveland, OH: Western Reserve Geriatric Education Center.

Anetzberger, G.J. (1997). Elderly adult survivors of family violence: Implications for clinical practice. *Violence Against Women, 3* (5), 499-514.

Anetzberger, G.J. (2000). Caregiving: Primary cause of elder abuse? *Generations, 24* (2), 46-51.

Anetzberger, G.J. (2001). Elder abuse identification and referral: The importance of screening tools and referral protocols. *Journal of Elder Abuse & Neglect, 13* (2), 3-22.

Anetzberger, G.J., Ejaz, F.K., Bass, D.M., & Nagpaul, K. (1999). *Abuse against older Ohioans in home and community based settings: Screening tools and referral protocol for service providers for stopping abuse against older Ohioans.* Cleveland, OH: The Benjamin Rose Institute.

Anetzberger, G.J., Korbin, J.E., & Tomita, S.K. (1996). Defining elder mistreatment in four groups across two generations. *Journal of Cross-Cultural Gerontology, 11,* 187-212.

Ansello, E.F. (1996). Causes and theories. In L.A. Baumhover & S.C. Beall (Eds.), *Abuse, neglect, and exploitation of older persons: Strategies for assessment and intervention* (pp. 9-29). Baltimore: Health Professions Press.

Archstone Foundation. (1998). *Understanding and combating elder abuse in minority communities: An exploration of the growing epidemic of elder abuse.* Long Beach, CA: Author.

Baker, A.A. (1975). Granny-battering. *Modern Geriatrics, 5* (8), 20-24.

Bass, D.M., Anetzberger, G.J., Ejaz, F.K., & Nagpaul, K. (2001). Screening tools and referral protocol for stopping abuse against older Ohioans: A guide for service providers. *Journal of Elder Abuse & Neglect, 13* (2), 23-38.

Blakely, B.E., & Dolon, R. (1991). The relative contributions of occupation groups in the discovery and treatment of elder abuse and neglect. *Journal of Gerontological Social Work, 17* (1/2), 183-199.

Blanton, P.G. (1989). Zen and the art of adult protective services: In search of a unified view. *Journal of Elder Abuse & Neglect, 1* (1), 27-34.

Blenkner, M., Bloom, M., Nielson, M., & Weber, R. (1974). *Final report: Protective services for older people, findings from the Benjamin Rose Institute study.* Cleveland OH: The Benjamin Rose Institute.

Block, M.R., & Sinnott, J.D. (Eds.) (1979). *The battered elder syndrome: An exploratory study.* College Park, MD: University of Maryland, Center of Aging.

Brandl, B., & Raymond, J. (1997). Unrecognized elder abuse victims: Older abused women. *Journal of Case Management, 6* (2), 62-68.

Bristowe, E., & Collins, J.B. (1989). Family mediated abuse of non-institutionalized elder men and women living in British Columbia. *Journal of Elder Abuse & Neglect, 1* (1), 45-54.

Brody, S.J. (1977). Resources for long-term care in the community. In E.M. Brody (Ed.), *Long-term care of older people: A practical guide* (pp. 59-83). New York: Human Sciences.

Brown, A.S. (1989). A survey on elder abuse at one native American tribe. *Journal of Elder Abuse & Neglect, 1* (2), 17-37.

Burr, J.J. (1971). Protective services for older adults: A demonstration project. *Welfare in Review, 9,* 1-6.

Burston, G.R. (1975). Granny-battering. *British Medical Journal, 3* (5983), 592.

Butler, R.N. (1975). *Why survive? Being old in America.* New York: Harper & Row.

Callahan, J.J., Jr. (1988). Elder abuse: Some questions for policymakers. *The Gerontologist, 28* (4), 453-458.

Carp, F.M. (2000). *Elder abuse in the family: An interdisciplinary model for research.* New York: Springer Publishing Company.

Chang, J., & Moon, A. (1997). Korean American elderly's knowledge and perceptions of elder abuse: A qualitative analysis of cultural factors. *Journal of Multicultural Social Work, 6* (1/2), 139-154.

Clark, A.N.G, Mankikar, G.D., & Gray, I. (1975). Diogenes syndrome: A clinical study of gross neglect in old age. *The Lancet 1, 790,* 366-368.

Comijs, H.C., Penninx, B.W.J.H., Knipscheer, K.P.M., & VanTilburg, W. (1999). Psychological distress in victims of elder mistreatment: The effects of social support and coping. *Journal of Gerontology: Psychological Sciences, 54B* (4), 240-245.

Comijs, H.C., Pot, A.M., Smit, J.H., Bouter, L.M., & Jonker, C. (1998). Elder abuse in the community: Prevalence and consequences. *Journal of the American Geriatrics Society, 46,* 885-888.

Cook-Daniels, L. (1997). Lesbian, gay male, bisexual and transgendered elders: Elder abuse and neglect issues. *Journal of Elder Abuse & Neglect, 9* (2), 35-49.

Coyne, A.C., Petenza, M., & Berbig, L.J. (1996). Abuse in families coping with dementia. *Aging, 367,* 93-95.

Daniels, R.S., Baumhover, L.A., & Clark-Daniels, C.L. (1989). Physicians' mandatory reporting of elder abuse. *The Gerontologist, 29* (3), 321-327.

Dolon, R., & Blakely, B. (1989). Elder abuse and neglect: A study of adult protective service workers in the United States. *Journal of Elder Abuse & Neglect, 1* (3), 31-49.

Dolon, R., & Hendricks, J.E. (1989). An exploratory study comparing attitudes and practices of police officers and social service providers in elder abuse and neglect cases. *Journal of Elder Abuse & Neglect, 1* (1), 75-90.

Douglass, R.L., Hickey, T., & Noel, C. (1980). *A study of maltreatment of the elderly and other vulnerable adults.* Ann Arbor: University of Michigan, Institute of Gerontology.

Faulkner, L.R. (1982). Mandating the reporting of suspected cases of elder abuse: An inappropriate, ineffective, and ageist response to the abuse of elder adults. *Family Law Quarterly, 16,* 69-91.

Floyd, J. (1984). Collecting data on abuse of the elderly. *Journal of Gerontology Nursing, 10* (12), 11-15.

Fredriksen, K.I. (1989). Adult protective services: Changes with the introduction of mandatory reporting. *Journal of Elder Abuse & Neglect, 1* (2), 59-70.

Fulmer, T.T., & O'Malley, T.A. (1987). *Inadequate care of the elderly: A health care perspective on abuse and neglect.* New York: Springer Publishing Company.

Gelles, R. (1991, May). *Review of theoretical models in family violence.* Paper presented at the National Institute on Aging Family Conflict and Elder Abuse Workshop. Bethesda, MD.

Gelles, R.J., & Cornell, C.P. (1985). *Intimate violence in families.* Newbury Park, CA: Sage.

Gilbert, D.A. (1986). The ethics of mandatory elder abuse reporting statutes. *Advances in Nursing Science, 8* (2), 51-62.

Gioglio, G.R., & Blakemore, P. (1983). *Elder abuse in New Jersey: The knowledge and experience of abuse among older New Jerseyans.* Trenton, NJ: New Jersey Department of Human Resources and New Jersey Department of Community Affairs.

Griffin, L.W. (1994). Elder maltreatment among rural African-Americans. *Journal of Elder Abuse & Neglect, 6* (1), 1-27.

Grossman, S. F. & Lundy, M. (2003). Use of domestic violence services across race and ethnicity by women aged 55 and older. *Violence Against Women, 9* (12), 1442-1452.

Harris, S.B. (1996). For better or for worse: Spouse abuse grown old. *Journal of Elder Abuse & Neglect, 8* (1), 1-33.

Horowitz, G., & Estes, C. (1971). *Protective services for the aged.* Washington, DC: US Department of Health, Education, and Welfare.

Huber, R., Netting, F.E., & Kautz, J.R. (1996). Differences in types of complaints and how they were resolved by local Long-Term Care Ombudsmen operating out of area agencies on aging. *Journal of Applied Gerontology, 15* (1), 87-101.

Hudson, M.F. (1986). Elder neglect and abuse: Current research. In K.A. Pillemer & R.S. Wolf (Eds.), *Elder abuse: Conflict in the family* (pp. 125-166). Dover, MA: Auburn House.

Hudson, M.F. (1991). Elder mistreatment: A taxonomy with definitions by Delphi. *Journal of Elder Abuse & Neglect, 3* (2), 1-20.

Hudson, M.F., Armachain, W.D., Beasley, C.M., & Carlson, J.R. (1998). Elder abuse: Two native American views. *The Gerontologist, 38* (5), 538-548.

Hudson, M.F., Beasley, C., Benedict, R.H., Carlson, J.R., Craig, B.F., Herman, C., & Mason, S.C. (2000). Elder abuse: Some Caucasian-American views. *Journal of Elder Abuse & Neglect, 12* (1), 89-114.

Hudson, M.F., & Carlson, J.R. (1999). Elder abuse: Its meaning to Caucasians, African Americans, and Native Americans. In T. Tatara (Ed.), *Understanding elder abuse in minority populations* (pp. 187-204). Philadelphia: Brunner/Mazel.

Hwalek, M. (1987). *Elder abuse demonstration program: Final report.* Springfield: Illinois Department on Aging.

Johnson, T. (1986). Critical issues in the definition of elder mistreatment. In K.A. Pillemer & R.S. Wolf (Eds.), *Elder abuse: Conflict in the family* (pp. 167-196). Dover, MA: Auburn House.

Johnson, T. (1991). *Elder mistreatment: Deciding who is at risk.* Westport, CT: Greenwood.

Johnson, T.F. (1999). Ethical issues: In whose best interest? In T.F. Johnson (Ed.), *Handbook on ethical issues in aging* (pp. 1-23). Westport, CT: Greenwood Press.

Jones, J. (1988). Emergency department protocol for the diagnosis and evaluation of geriatric abuse. *Annals of Emergency Medicine, 17,* 1006-1015.

Jones, J.S. (1990). Geriatric abuse and neglect. In G. Bosker, G.R. Schwartz, J.S. Jones, & M. Sequeira (Eds.), *Geriatric emergency medicine* (pp. 533-542). St. Louis: C.V. Mosby.

Kapp, M.B. (1995). Elder mistreatment: Legal interventions and policy uncertainties. *Behavioral Sciences and the Law, 13,* 365-380.

Kivela, S., Kongas-Saviaro, P., Kesti, E., Pahkala, K., & Ijas, M. (1992). Abuse in old age–Epidemiological data from Finland. *Journal of Elder Abuse & Neglect, 4*(3), 1-18.

Kosberg, J.I., & Garcia, J.L. (Eds.). (1995). Elder abuse: International and cross-cultural perspectives. *Journal of Elder Abuse & Neglect, 6* (3/4).

Kosberg, J.I., & Nahmiash, D. (1996). Characteristics of victims and perpetrators and milieus of abuse and neglect. In L.A. Baumhover & S.C. Beall (Eds.), *Abuse, ne-*

glect, and exploitation of older persons: Strategies for assessment and intervention (pp. 31-49). Baltimore: Health Professions Press.

Krassen Maxwell, E., & Maxwell, R.J. (1992). Insults to the body civil: Mistreatment of elderly in two Plain Indian tribes. *Journal of Cross-Cultural Gerontology, 7*, 3-23.

Lachs, M.S., & Pillemer, K. (1995). Abuse and neglect of elderly persons. *The New England Journal of Medicine, 332* (7), 437-443.

Lachs, M.S., Williams, C., O'Brien, S., Hurst, L., & Horwitz, R. (1997). Risk factors for reported elder abuse and neglect: A nine-year observational cohort study. *The Gerontologist, 37* (4), 469-474.

Lau, E.E., & Kosberg, J.I. (1979). Abuse of the elderly by informal care providers. *Aging, 299-300*, 10-15.

Macolini, R.M. (1995). Elder abuse policy: Considerations in research and legislation. *Behavioral Sciences and the Law, 13*, 349-363.

McLaughlin, C. (1988). "Doing good": A worker's perspective. *Public Welfare, 46* (2), 29-32.

McLaughlin, J.S., Nickell, J.P., & Gill, L. (1980). An epidemiological investigation on elderly abuse in Southern Maine and New Hampshire. In US Senate Special Committee on Aging & US House Select Committee on Aging, *Elder abuse: Joint hearing* (pp. 111-147). Washington, DC: US Government Printing Office.

Mendelson, M.A. (1974). *Tender loving greed: How the incredibly lucrative nursing home "industry" is exploiting America's old people and defrauding us all.* New York: Alfred A. Knopf.

Mixson, P.M. (1995). An adult protective services perspective. *Journal of Elder Abuse & Neglect, 7* (2/3), 69-87.

Moon, A., & Williams, O. (1993). Perceptions of elder abuse and help-seeking patterns among African-American, Caucasian American, and Korean-American elderly women. *The Gerontologist, 33* (3), 386-395.

Moon, A., Tomita, S. K. & Jung-Kamei, S. (2001). Elder mistreatment among four Asian American groups: An exploratory study on tolerance, victim blaming and attitudes toward third-party intervention. *Journal of Gerontological Social Work, 36* (1/2), 153-169.

Nadien, M.B. (1995). Elder violence (maltreatment) in domestic settings: Some theory and research. In L.L. Adler & F.L. Denmark (Eds.), *Violence and the prevention of violence* (pp. 177-190). Westport, CT: Praeger.

Nagpaul, K. (1997). Elder abuse among Asian Indians: Traditional versus modern perspectives. *Journal of Elder Abuse & Neglect, 9* (2), 77-92.

National Center on Elder Abuse. (1997, November). *Reporting of elder abuse in domestic settings* (Elder Abuse Information Series No. 3). Washington, DC: Author.

National Center on Elder Abuse. (1998, September). *The national elder abuse incidence study.* Washington, DC: Author.

National Center on Elder Abuse (1999, March). *Types of elder abuse in domestic settings* (Elder Abuse Information Series No. 1). Washington, DC: Author.

National Research Council (2003). Elder mistreatment: Abuse, neglect, and exploitation in an aging America. Washington, DC: The National Academies Press.

Nerenberg, L. (1994). *Older battered women: Integrating aging and domestic violence services.* Washington, DC: National Center on Elder Abuse.

Ogg, J., & Bennett, G.C.J. (1992). Elder abuse in Britain. *British Medical Journal, 305*, 998-999.

Ohio Department of Human Services. (1996). *SFY 1996 Adult protective services fact sheet.* Columbus, OH: Author.

Ohio Department of Job and Family Services. (2000). *Adult protective services fact sheet SFY 2000.* Columbus, OH: Author.

O'Malley, H., Segars, H., Perez, R., Mitchell, V., & Knuepfel, G.M. (1979). *Elder abuse in Massachusetts: A survey of professionals and para-professionals.* Boston: Legal Research and Services for the Elderly.

O'Neill, V. (1965). Protecting older people. *Public Welfare, 23* (2), 119-127.

Osgood, N.J., & Manetta, A.A. (2000-2001). Abuse and suicidal issues in older women. *OMEGA, 42*(1), 71-81.

Otto, J.M. (2000). The role of adult protective services in addressing abuse. *Generations, 24* (11), 33-38.

Payne, B.K., & Kovic, R. (1995). An empirical examination of the characteristics, consequences, and causes of elder abuse in nursing homes. *Journal of Elder Abuse & Neglect, 7* (4), 61-74.

Phillips, L.R. (1983). Abuse and neglect of the frail elderly at home: An exploration of theoretical relationships. *Journal of Advanced Nursing, 8,* 379-392.

Phillips, L.R. (1986). Theoretical explanations of elder abuse: Competing hypotheses and unresolved issues. In K.A. Pillemer & R.S. Wolf (Eds.), *Elder abuse: Conflict in the family* (pp. 197-217). Dover, MA: Auburn House.

Pillemer, K. (1985, October). *Domestic violence against the elderly.* Paper presented at the Surgeon General's Workshop on Violence and Public Health, Leesburg, VA.

Pillemer, K., & Finkelhor, D. (1988). The prevalence of elder abuse: A random sample survey. *The Gerontologist, 28,* 51-57.

Pillemer, K., & Prescott, D. (1989). Psychological effects of elder abuse: A research note. *Journal of Elder Abuse & Neglect, 1* (1), 65-74.

Podnieks, E. (1992). National survey on abuse of the elderly in Canada. *Journal of Elder Abuse & Neglect, 4* (1/2), 5-58.

Quinn, M.J., & Tomita, S.K. (1997). *Elder abuse and neglect: Causes, diagnosis, and intervention strategies* (2nd ed.). New York: Springer Publishing Company.

Ramsey-Klawsnik, H. (1991). Elder sexual abuse: Preliminary findings. *Journal of Elder Abuse & Neglect, 3* (3), 73-90.

Rathbone-McCuan, E., & Hashimi, J. (1982). *Isolated elders: Health and social intervention.* Rockville, MD: Aspen.

Regan, J.J. (1978). Intervention through adult protective services programs. *The Gerontologist, 18* (3), 250-254.

Regan, J.J. (1990). *The aged client and the law.* New York: Columbia University Press.

Reis, M., & Nahmiash, D. (1998). Validation of the indicators of abuse (IOA) screen. *The Gerontologist, 38* (4), 471-480.

Rosenblatt, D.E., Cho, K.H., & Durance, P.W. (1996). Reporting mistreatment of elder adults: The role of physicians. *Journal of the American Geriatrics Society, 44,* 65-70.

Roybal, E.R. (1991, May). Elder abuse: America's hidden crisis. *CARING Magazine, 10* (5), 22-24.

Salend, E., Kane, R.A., Satz, M., & Pynoos, J. (1984). Elder abuse reporting: Limitations of statutes. *The Gerontologist, 24* (1), 61-69.

Sanchez, Y.M. (1999). Elder mistreatment in Mexican American communities: The Nevada and Michigan experiences. In T. Tatara (Ed.), *Understanding elder abuse in minority populations* (pp. 67-77). Philadelphia: Brunner/Mazel.

Schene, P., & Ward, S.F. (1988). The vexing problem of elder abuse: The relevance of the child protection experience. *Public Welfare, 46* (2), 14-21.

Sengstock, M.C., & Liang, J. (1982). *Identifying and characterizing elder abuse.* Detroit: Wayne State University, Institute of Gerontology.

Simmelink, K. (1996). Lessons learned from three elderly sexual assault survivors. *Journal of Emergency Nursing, 22,* 619-621.

Stannard, C.I. (1973). Old folks and dirty work: The social conditions for patient abuse in a nursing home. *Social Problems, 20* (3), 329-342.

Stein, K.F. (1991). A national agenda for elder abuse and neglect research: Issues and recommendations. *Journal of Elder Abuse & Neglect, 3* (3), 91-108.

Stein, K.F. (1991, September). *Working with abused and neglected elders in minority populations: A synthesis of research.* Washington, DC: National Aging Resource Center on Elder Abuse.

Steinmetz, S.K. (1988). *Duty bound: Elder abuse and family care.* Newbury Park, CA: Sage.

Strauss, W., & Howe, N. (1991). *Generations: The history of America's future, 1584-2069.* New York: William Morrow.

Tatara, T. (1995, May). *An analysis of state laws addressing elder abuse, neglect, and exploitation.* Washington, DC: National Center on Elder Abuse.

Tatara, T. (1996, June). *Elder abuse: Questions and answers.* Washington, DC: National Center on Elder Abuse.

Tatara, T. (Ed.). (1997). Elder abuse in minority populations. *Journal of Elder Abuse & Neglect, 9* (2).

Tatara, T. (Ed.). (1999). *Understanding elder abuse in minority populations.* Philadelphia: Brunner/Mazel.

Tatara, T., & Kuzmeskus, L. (1997). *Summaries of statistical data on elder abuse in domestic settings for FY 95 and FY 96.* Washington, DC: National Center on Elder Abuse.

Teaster, P. B. (2003). A response to the abuse of vulnerable adults: The 2000 survey of state adult protective services. Washington, DC: National Center on Elder Abuse.

Thobaben, M. (1989). State elder/adult abuse and protection laws. In R. Filinson & S.R. Ingman (Eds.), *Elder abuse: Practice and policy* (pp. 138-152). New York: Human Services Press.

Tomita, S. (1994). The consideration of cultural factors in the research of elder mistreatment with an in-depth look at the Japanese. *Journal of Cross-Cultural Gerontology, 9,* 39-52.

Townsend, C. (1971). *Old age: The last segregation.* New York: Grossman.

Tueth, M.J. (2000). Exposing financial exploitation of impaired elderly persons. *American Journal of Geriatric Psychiatry, 8* (2), 104-111.

United Nations Economic and Social Council. (2002, February 25-March 1). *Abuse of older persons: Recognizing and responding to abuse of older persons in a global context.* Document of the Commission for Social Development presented at the Second World Assembly on Aging, New York, NY.

US Department of Health and Human Services. (1992). *Report from the Secretary's Task Force on Elder Abuse.* Washington, DC: Author.

US General Accounting Office. (1991). *Elder abuse: Effectiveness of reporting laws and other factors.* Washington, DC: Author.

US House Select Committee of Aging. (1990). *Elder abuse: A decade of shame and inaction* (Comm. Pub. No. 101-752). Washington, DC: US Government Printing Office.

US House Select Committee on Aging. (1980). *Elder abuse: The hidden problem, A briefing, June 23, 1979, Boston, MA*. Washington, DC: US Government Printing Office.

US House Select Committee on Aging & US House Science and Technology Subcommittee on Domestic, International, Scientific Planning, Analysis and Cooperation. (1978). *Domestic violence*. Washington, DC: US Government Printing Office.

US Senate Special Committee on Aging. (1977). *Protective services for the elderly: A working paper*. Washington, DC: US Government Printing Office.

University of New Hampshire. (1986). *Elder abuse and neglect: Recommendations from the Research Conference on Elder Abuse and Neglect*. Durham, NH: Author.

Wasser, E. (1971). Protective practice in serving the mentally impaired aged. *Social Casework, 52* (8), 510-522.

Watson, M.M. (1995). *Silent suffering: Elder abuse in America: Conference summary and recommendations for the 1995 White House Conference on Aging*. Unpublished manuscript.

Wiehe, V.R. (1998). *Understanding family violence: Treating and preventing partner, child, sibling, and elder abuse*. Thousand Oaks, CA: Sage.

Wilber, K.H., & Reynolds, S.L. (1996). Introducing a framework for defining financial abuse of the elderly. *Journal of Elder Abuse & Neglect, 8* (2), 61-80.

Wolf, R.S. (1988). Elder abuse: Ten years later. *Journal of the American Geriatrics Society, 36* (8), 758-762.

Wolf, R.S. (1997). Elder abuse and neglect: An update. *Reviews in Clinical Gerontology, 7*, 177-182.

Wolf, R.S., Godkin, M.A., & Pillemer, K.A. (1984). *Elder abuse and neglect: Final report from Three Model Projects*. Worcester, MA: University of Massachusetts Medical Center, University Center on Aging.

Wolf, R.S., Godkin, M.A., & Pillemer, K.A. (1986). Maltreatment of the elderly: A comparative analysis. *Pride Institute Journal of Long Term Home Health Care, 5*, 10-17.

Wolf, R.S., & Nerenberg, L. (1994, December). *Compendium ·of products on elder abuse from grants funded under Title IV of the Older Americans Act Administration on Aging*. Worcester, MA: National Committee for the Prevention of Elder Abuse.

Wynkoop, T.F., & Gerstein, L.H. (1993). Staff burnout in adult protective services work. In B. Byers & J.E. Hendricks (Eds.), *Adult protective services: Research and practice* (pp. 191-229). Springfield, IL: Charles C Thomas.

Zborowsky, E. (1985). Developments in protective services: A challenge for social workers. *Journal of Gerontological Social Work, 8* (3/4), 71-83.

Clinical Management of Elder Abuse: General Considerations

Georgia J. Anetzberger, PhD, ACSW, LISW

SUMMARY. Clinical management of elder abuse situations involves five steps: detection, assessment, planning, intervention, and follow-up. Although each clinical discipline brings a unique set of knowledge, skills, and perspectives to completing the steps, there are general considerations that universally apply in successfully identifying and treating the problem. These general considerations are described, with particular attention given to the intent behind actions, strategies for step accomplishment, and issues likely to emerge. *[Article copies available for a fee from The Haworth Document Delivery Service: 1-800-HAWORTH. E-mail address: <docdelivery@haworthpress.com> Website: <http://www.HaworthPress.com> © 2005 by The Haworth Press, Inc. All rights reserved.]*

KEYWORDS. Clinical management in elder abuse, abuse detection, assessment, case planning, intervention and follow-up

There are any number of ways that clinicians encounter elder abuse situations. In most instances, encounter will not be during actual abuse occurrence. Only rarely, for example, will clinicians be present when acts of physical abuse or violations of rights happen. Physicians and nurses

Georgia J. Anetzberger is Research Associate, Visiting Nurse Association, Healthcare Partners of Ohio, Cleveland, Ohio.

[Haworth co-indexing entry note]: "Clinical Management of Elder Abuse: General Considerations." Anetzberger, Georgia J. Co-published simultaneously in *Clinical Gerontologist* (The Haworth Press, Inc.) Vol. 28, No. 1/2, 2005, pp. 27-41; and: *The Clinical Management of Elder Abuse* (ed: Georgia J. Anetzberger) The Haworth Press, Inc., 2005, pp. 27-41. Single or multiple copies of this article are available for a fee from The Haworth Document Delivery Service [1-800-HAWORTH, 9:00 a.m. - 5:00 p.m. (EST). E-mail address: docdelivery@haworthpress.com].

typically are not around to witness an elderly husband hit his wife, even when this has been a pattern for decades and health professionals are seen on a regular basis by the couple. Similarly, attorneys and social workers seldom are present when a caregiving daughter denies visitors to or opens the mail of her dependant parents, even when reports of this problem have surfaced among neighbors in the past. Much more common is for clinicians to encounter elder abuse situations in the aftermath of abuse occurrence, or alternatively to come across older people whose characteristics and circumstances suggest the possibility of elder abuse in the future. Accordingly, the first step in the clinical management of elder abuse situations involves detecting the problem. The other steps in order are: assessment, planning, intervention, and follow-up. The sections below discuss each of the five steps in elder abuse clinical management, with attention given to answering several related questions: What is the intent of this step in clinical management? Who is targeted? What tasks are undertaken? What issues are likely to emerge? Are particular strategies or approaches considered? Are any instruments or protocols employed?

DETECTION

The purpose of detection is for clinicians to decide whether or not elder abuse is known or suspected in a situation involving an older person who is a current client or has been referred for evaluation or service provision. Elder abuse is "known" if it is personally observed or if it is reported by the victim or some other person capable of having that knowledge. Elder abuse is "suspected" through the identification of signs which represent the consequence of abuse occurrence. Signs suggest the probability of elder abuse. However, because they can have other origins, signs alone seldom offer conclusiveness that elder abuse has taken place. Illustrations of signs include broken bones for physical abuse or dehydration for physical neglect. Yet, broken bones also can result from accidental falls and dehydration from acute illnesses.

Deciding whether or not elder abuse is known or suspected is a prerequisite for reporting the problem to authorities charged with its investigation. Most state adult protective services or elder abuse reporting laws use these criteria for case referral. More than four-fifths of the states have mandatory reporting laws that require health and social service professionals to report elder abuse. Those professionals most frequently identified in the laws as mandatory reporters are social workers, physicians, law enforcement officers, psychologists and nurses (Tatara, 1995; Teaster, 2003).

Even when elder abuse is neither known nor suspected as a result of clinical detection, the process might reveal risk factors for abuse occurrence. Risk factors are characteristics that have been found associated with elder abuse through research on the subject (Anetzberger, 2001). The identification of risk factors indicates the possibility of abuse occurrence. The problem could happen in the future. Examples of physical abuse risk factors include financial dependence and substance abuse for an adult son residing with his elderly mother. Examples of physical neglect risk factors include functional impairment and dependence for an elderly father and caregiver stress and burden for the adult daughter who provides him with caregiving assistance. Risk factors are like "red flags." They serve to alert clinicians and remind them to be on the watch for examples and signs of elder abuse.

Detecting elder abuse usually requires awareness of the problem and a high level of suspicion (Abyad, 1996). These qualities must be sustained across time, settings, and client contexts. Otherwise, elder abuse situations will be missed (Phillips, 1983). Indications of abuse occurrence can come from observing or interviewing clients in clinical settings, such as professional offices, hospitals, and community-based services. However, the problem is most likely to reveal itself by visiting older people in their own homes. It is here that the consequences of abuse occurrence are often evidenced in a mosaic of physical and behavioral indicators, from accumulated waste as a result of elder incapacity for living alone to fear as a result of victim/perpetrator conflict. Because with time these indicators become part of life's design, they are difficult to hide. Consequently, it is little wonder that the professionals most likely to detect and report elder abuse are those who typically see clients at home (Blakely & Dolon, 1991).

The likelihood of detecting elder abuse increases the wider the net of observation and inquiry made by clinicians. In this regard, both the victim and perpetrator should be interviewed, and interviewed both together and separately. Group interviews enable the clinician to see victim/perpetrator interaction. Separate interviews facilitate individual candor and enable comparison of accounts.

It is important to recognize that the clinicians' perspective of victims and perpetrators or their personal values may interfere with abuse detection. For example, clinicians may overlook or misinterpret elder abuse situations where the older person's disturbing behaviors are seen as provocative or the caregiving perpetrator's attitude is one of cooperation or conciliation (Phillips & Rempusheski, 1986). Moreover, strong beliefs on individual privacy or family sanctity may cause clinicians to ignore elder abuse situations. Other barriers to abuse detection can exist for clinicians as well, including lack of understanding about the problem and a narrow focus on professional responsibilities because of time pressures or personal attitude.

Nonetheless, it is not just clinicians with barriers to abuse detection. Barriers can exist with the victims and perpetrators themselves (Aldeman, Siddiqui, & Foldi, 1998). For instance, victims may deny abuse occurrence. They may be unaware of it because of cognitive or other impairment. They also may redefine it as something other than elder abuse on the basis of cultural or family background. Likewise, perpetrators may see elder abuse as necessary action to protect victims, for example, in the inappropriate use of chemical or physical restraints with dependent older people who are confused and wander. They may consider elder abuse as just punishment when victims are combative and assaultive toward them or when there has been a history of family violence, with the victim assuming the perpetrator role in earlier times. Perpetrators also may attempt to hide abuse occurrence or convince victims of its necessity.

Several instruments have been developed to improve and systematize the elder abuse detection process. Typically called screening or risk assessment tools, their intent is to identify abused elders, those at risk of abuse, or both (Wolf, 2000a). Few such tools are universally accepted, and most have not been tested for reliability or validity. However, they are important in the clinical management of elder abuse because of their ability to aid in abuse detection (National Research Council, 2003). In this regard, screening and risk assessment tools insure that manifestations and risk factors for elder abuse are not missed. They formalize the process of observation and inquiry, and they provide a database for research (Sengstock, Hwalek, & Moshier, 1986; Fulmer & O'Malley, 1987; Fulmer & Gould, 1996; Neale, Hwalek, Scott, Sengstock, & Stahl, 1991; Marshall, Benton, & Brazier, 2000; Wolf, 2000).

Minimally, screening and risk assessment tools should include questions on demographics, common signs and risk factors for each abuse form, and degree of endangerment (Aravanis et al., 1993). Structurally these tools range from narrative guidelines to checklists, from comprehensive catalogues to abbreviated indices. Some tools are geared to use in particular settings, like hospitals or adult protective service agencies. Others relate to select professionals, like physicians or nurses. Examples of elder abuse screening and risk assessment tools include the following: Harborview Medical Center Elder Abuse and Neglect Written Protocol for Identification and Assessment (Tomita, 1982); Health, Attitudes, Living Arrangements, and Finances (H.A.L.F.) (Ferguson & Beck, 1983); Protective Services Risk Assessment (Daiches, 1983); Sengstock-Hwalek Comprehensive Index of Elder Abuse (Sengstock, Hwalek, & Moshier, 1986); Geriatric Abuse Protocol (Jones et al., 1988); Elder Mistreatment Detection Protocol Package (Johnson, 1991); American Medical Association Diagnostic and Treatment Guidelines on Elder Abuse and Neglect (American Medical Association, 1992); Florida and Illinois adult protective services risk assessment tools (Goodrich, 1997); Indicators of Abuse (Reis & Nahmiash, 1998); and Actual/Suspected/Risk of Abuse Tools (Bass et al., 2000).

ASSESSMENT

The presence of elder abuse signs or risk factors indicates the need for a more thorough assessment. Conversely, a thorough assessment may be required in order to reveal elder abuse signs and risk factors (Gray-Vickrey, 2000). The purpose of the assessment process is to evaluate the person and situation of victim and perpetrator in order to determine: need for assistance, immediacy of need, available resources to assist, and identified priorities for receipt of assistance. Assessment involves the collection of information from multiple sources, including the victim, caregiver or perpetrator, other family members, and collaterals (All, 1994). The information is obtained through various mechanisms, such as interviews, clinical testing, and background checks.

Particularly important, and potentially difficult, are assessment interviews. They are best approached recognizing and respecting the "5 Ps" of interviewing in general: privacy, pacing, planning, pitch, and punctuality (Villamore & Bergman, 1981). Moreover, consideration for individual rights and preferences is critical, if the clinician expects client movement from assessment to planning and intervention in clinical management. Resistance to help can, and usually will, emerge from victims and perpetrators when little empathy is expressed for personal struggles, wishes are ignored, individual strengths are minimized, and interventions are rushed.

An assessment represents an organized approach for collecting information about people and their circumstances. Its importance lies in its ability to improve the accuracy of problem identification, provide information for planning interventions, and avoid the inappropriate use of services. Minimally an assessment of elder abuse victims and perpetrators and their situations should cover: physical health problems, mental and cognitive status changes, functional limitations, financial and environmental issues, recent family or life crises, and diminished social resources. In addition, the nature of the elder abuse should be evaluated, including its forms, frequency, intent, severity, and longevity. Finally, Quinn and Tomita (1997) recommend inquiry about a typical day and care or assistance expectations as part of the assessment process. Instruments employed during assessment depend upon the specific conditions being evaluated, such as the activities of daily living scale for functional limitations and Mini-Mental Status Examination for cognitive impairment. In some instances, assessment and related instrument use will be layered, with problem confirmation at one level suggesting the need for more in-depth explanation. For example, identification of cognitive decline using the Dementia Scale may indicate the need for a comprehensive neuropsychological evaluation (Breckman & Adelman, 1988).

PLANNING

The purpose of the planning step in clinical management is to delineate a course of action based upon assessment findings. This is not easy. Sometimes clinicians err in their associations between problem identification and intervention decision (Phillips & Rempusheski, 1985). This can happen because they fail to understand underlying abuse etiology or to unravel the consequences of abuse occurrence, both of which help facilitate sound intervention selection (Adelman & Breckman, 1995).

Other times, the paradigm clinicians use to guide action is inappropriate (Phillips, 1988). Nerenberg (2000) discusses several paradigms or approaches used to address elder abuse. They include: protective services, elder rights, domestic-violence, criminal justice, and multidisciplinary team. Other observers offer additional paradigms, such as family-oriented (Rathbone-McCuan, Travis, & Voyles, 1983), social network (Hooyman, 1982), environmental press (Ansello, King, & Taler, 1986), inadequate care (Fulmer & O'Malley, 1987), and systems (Segal & Iris, 1989). Each paradigm or approach tends to have its own philosophy, intervention strategies, and preferred services or other resources. Given the complexity of elder abuse as a problem and as it manifests itself in individual instances, it is probable that every approach fits some abuse situations and that multiple approaches may apply in select ones.

Unfortunately, professional orientation, agency policy, personal bias, or ignorance may undermine appropriate paradigm selection, making choice automatic rather than a thoughtful consideration of the dynamics of the elder abuse situation in question.

Two goals are employed in planning elder abuse interventions: preserving victim autonomy and promoting victim safety. Although sometimes at odds with one another, these goals are primary in clinical management (Lachs & Pillemer, 1995). Achieving them is often dependent upon two factors. The first concerns the ability and willingness of the victim and perpetrator to accept assistance. Case planning will be different for competent, consenting clients than it will be for competent, nonconsenting or incompetent ones (Villamore & Bergman, 1981). The second factor surrounds the quality of the intervention resources themselves. The adequacy and effectiveness of specific treatments, services, or benefits can affect client outcome and therefore influence case planning. In this light, it is noteworthy that evaluative research on elder abuse interventions has been minimal, and when specific programs or services have been tested, they frequently have not been shown effective (Wilber & Nielsen, 2002, Fulmer & Anetzberger, 1995).

INTERVENTION

The intervention step in clinical management involves the application of services, laws, and clinical procedures to treat the consequences of elder abuse or prevent occurrence or reoccurrence of the problem. It surrounds the implementation of the case plan.

Elder abuse service interventions have been organized in several different ways. For example, Collins (1982) arranges help for victims by service type: core (like assessment and counseling), emergency (including temporary financial support and emergency shelter), legal and financial (such as power of attorney and banking options), medical and personal care (like mental health services and home health care), home support and housing (including foster care and home repair), and social support (such as day care and support groups). Podnieks (1985) describes three levels of prevention: primary (like legislation and advocacy), secondary (including medical treatment for injuries and protective services), and tertiary (such as substance abuse counseling and anger management). Baumhover, Beall, and Pieroni (1990) divide interventions by targeted group (i.e., victim, abuser, or community) and response level (i.e., social policy, community, and professional). Quinn and

Tomita's (1997) organization of interventions considers time duration (i.e., crisis intervention, short-term, or long-term) and targeted person (i.e., victim or perpetrator). Finally, Anetzberger (2000) offers an integrative framework for elder abuse intervention that has three intersecting components: approach (i.e., protection, empowerment, or advocacy), target (i.e., victim-perpetrator dyad or family system), and basic intervention function (i.e., emergency response, support, rehabilitation, or prevention).

Research on specific service or program interventions used in elder abuse situations suggests variation by abuse form and targeted person. For example, Sengstock, Hwalek, and Petrone (1989) found that victims of confinement/deprivation and financial abuse received the most services and victims of physical abuse the least. Services almost exclusively went to the victims; very few went to the perpetrators. Moreover, choice of service to victims mirrored that extended to frail older people in general, and reflected types of services found in social work and home care settings. In studying service delivery to competent, self-neglecting elders in Wisconsin, Vinton (1991) found that typically only one service was offered to each victim, although other services existed in the community. Additionally, among 25 different services planned for 227 victims, the most common were: information and referral, supportive health care, case management, home health care, mental health services, home-delivered meals, and counseling. In a comparison study of physically abusing caregivers and noncaregiving abusers, Vinton (1992) discovered that few perpetrators were offered any services. However, when services were offered, caregiving abusers received more than noncaregiving abusers, even when the latter demonstrated greater need. Lastly, Nahmiash and Reis (2000) found that abuse victims were most likely to accept and benefit from concrete services, like medical care and homemaking, or empowerment strategies, like support groups and advocates. Perpetrators most accepted and benefited from individual counseling and education/training. Furthermore, in comparing victims and perpetrators, perpetrators both accepted and benefited from services more than victims.

Legal interventions to address elder abuse vary by state. However, nearly all states have available civil and criminal remedies as well as common law and law specific to elder abuse (Moskowitz, 1998). In Ohio, for example, criminal remedy exists in the abuse or neglect of an elderly or disabled person by a caretaker law, and civil remedy in the protective services law for adults, which exclusively considers abuse, neglect, or exploitation experienced by impaired persons age 60 years and older.

Situations of elder physical abuse also may be covered as statutory crimes under such laws as those dealing with assault and battery. However, it has been noted that tort law is deficient with respect to elder abuse in that it does not always consider the various abuse forms experienced by older adults nor does it always consider abuse consequences as legally actionable (Polisky, 1995). In Ohio, as elsewhere, financial abuse may be covered by laws addressing theft, fraud, or larceny, among others. In addition, the Ohio General Assembly enacted legislation a few years ago that provided greater penalty against those who violate select exploitation laws by victimizing either elderly adults or those with disabilities. Finally, protection for incompetent or incapacitated older adults is available through court appointment of surrogate decision-makers, such as guardians (Kapp, 1995; Moskowitz, 1998).

In Ohio, as in most states, the criminalization of elder abuse began in the late 1980s (Heisler, 1991; Stiegel, 1995). Prior to that, the emphasis was placed on assisting victims through a wide range of services and, if needed, through involuntary protective intervention or appointment of surrogate decision-making authority. The criminalization of elder abuse reflects many factors. These include the following: (1) the current preference in American society for punishment over rehabilitation in treating unacceptable behaviors; (2) the sometimes lack of success in dealing with elder abuse situations using services and civil remedies alone; (3) the ever-broadening definition of elder abuse, increasingly incorporating actions, like fraud and scams, traditionally approached through criminal justice measures; and (4) the entry of domestic violence advocates in the field of elder abuse, who historically have sought punishment for abusers as a preferred intervention. Nonetheless, with a problem as multidimensional as elder abuse, typically with complex relations between victims and perpetrators and limited available or acceptable care options for dependant older adults, intervention strategies often must combine the application of law with services, even in admittedly criminal cases. Otherwise, the arrest and imprisonment of the perpetrator may leave the victim without needed assistance, socially isolated, and at risk of self-neglect or institutionalization (Wolf, 2000b).

As an alternative to punishment or deterrence through the criminal justice system, victims or their families more and more are seeking restitution in the form of monetary damages from perpetrators, or those who fail to report their acts, through the civil justice system. Most such initiatives have focused on abuse or neglect in institutional settings, like nursing facilities (Jackson, 1999). However, this remedy can apply to domestic elder abuse as well (Payne, 2000).

It is not possible within the confines of this article to describe all the various clinical procedures that might be appropriate in elder abuse situations. Instead, some of the specific aims they should have are delineated. First, clinical procedures should address the victim's acute medical problems, including any injuries and untreated illnesses, and acute emotional problems resulting from elder abuse, including fear and anxiety (Miller & Veltkamp, 1998). Second, they should insure the victim's safety (Silverman & Hudson, 2000). This requires working with victims to identify ways to remain safe under particular circumstances (Brandl & Raymond, 1997; Hirsch, Stratton, & Loewyn, 1999). For some victims this may mean leaving their present residence to receive hospital treatment, emergency shelter, or nursing care. Third, clinical procedures should help victims regain the sense of efficacy and control that elder abuse eroded (Simmelink, 1996; Brandl, 2000). Key to empowering victims is giving them the information necessary to evaluate and decide among courses of actions. Empowerment also necessitates that clinicians relinquish decision-making to victims (unless the victims have been determined incompetent or incapacitated), and respecting choices made (even if the choices are different than those clinicians would have made themselves). Fourth, clinical procedures should serve to alleviate the underlying causes of elder abuse (Aravanis et al., 1993). In doing so, care must be taken to inform victims (along with perpetrators) about elder abuse, including its potential severity and effects.

FOLLOW-UP

Follow-up in elder abuse cases can have different purposes. Among the most important are evaluation of intervention effectiveness, reassessment of need, and situation monitoring to prevent abuse reoccurrence. In every instance, follow-up suggests the establishment of an ongoing relationship between victim (or perpetrator) and clinician, minimally characterized by a recognition that elder abuse and its effects typically do not end quickly or simply.

Elder abuse intervention requires a commitment to change on the part of the victim or perpetrator. Change is rarely easy, but it is particularly difficult in abuse situations of long duration and strong family bonds. Respecting client pace and degree of change can challenge clinicians not firmly rooted in principles for intervening on behalf of abused elders, such as those suggested by Anetzberger and Miller (1999). Hierarchically ranked, they are: freedom over safety, self-determination, participation in decision-making, least restrictive alternatives, primacy of the adult, confidentiality, benefit of doubt, do no harm, avoidance of blame, and maintenance of the family.

Elder abuse situations often require long-term or intermittent intervention before resolution (Quinn & Tomita, 1997). As a result, client dependency on the clinician and client inability to remain focused on the case plan are not uncommon practice issues. More troubling, however, are instances where clients refuse needed help. In Ohio during fiscal year 2003, 24 percent of older adults found in need of protective services because of substantiated abuse, neglect, or exploitation refused services (Ohio Department of Job and Family Services, 2003). An Illinois study on substantiated elder abuse reports to adult protective services discovered that victims who refuse services tend to have perpetrators who are substance abusers, have mental illness, or are financially dependent on the abusers (Neale, Hwalek, Goodrich, & Quinn, 1997).

Some victims lack the mental capacity to consent to services. In Ohio, and many other states, involuntary protective services can be offered through court order. In a national study of involuntary protective services, Duke (1993) found that among states which provide involuntary services, an average of 8 percent of adult protective services clients are served involuntarily.

Documentation is an essential component to elder abuse detection, assessment, planning, intervention, and follow-up (Rosenblatt, 1996). It provides an historical account, important for identifying trends. It enables clinicians to determine which practices are effective and which ones are not. It offers evidence that may be useful in legal actions. It is a reference for other clinicians who might follow, to facilitate coordinated care or service delivery. Documentation must be accurate and complete. It also should be timely and reflect the "regular course of business" during clinical contact. Finally, it may take multiple forms, from written records to photographs to clinical test results.

REFERENCES

Abyad, A. (1996, October). Elder abuse: Diagnosis, management, and prevention. *Medical Interface*, 97-101.

Adelman, R., & Breckman, R. (1995). Elder abuse and neglect. In *The Merck manual of geriatrics* (2nd ed.) (pp.1408-1416). Whitehouse Station, NJ: Merck.

Adelman, R.D., Siddiqui, H., & Foldi, N. (1998). Approaches to diagnosis and treatment of elder abuse and neglect. In M. Hersen & V.B. VanHasselt (Eds.), *Handbook of clinical geropsychology* (pp. 557-567). New York: Plenum Press.

All, A.C. (1994). A literature review: Assessment and intervention in elder abuse. *Journal of Gerontological Nursing, 20* (7), 25-32.

American Medical Association. (1992). *Diagnostic and treatment guidelines on elder abuse and neglect.* Chicago: Author.

Anetzberger, G.J. (2000). Caregiving: Primary source or elder abuse? *Generations, 24* (11), 46-51.

Anetzberger, G.J. (2001). Elder abuse identification and referral: The importance of screening tools and referral protocols. *Journal of Elder Abuse & Neglect, 13* (2), 3-22.

Anetzberger, G.J., & Miller, C.A. (1999). Impaired psychosocial function: Elder abuse and neglect. In C.A. Miller, *Nursing care of older adults: Theory & practice* (3rd ed.) (pp. 612-653). Philadelphia: Lippincott.

Ansello, E.F., King, N.R., & Taler, G. (1986). The environmental press model: A theoretical framework for intervention in elder abuse. In K.A. Pillemer & R.S. Wolf (Eds.), *Elder abuse: Conflict in the family* (pp. 314-330). Dover, MA: Auburn House.

Aravanis, S.C., Adelman, R.D., Breckman, R., Fulmer, T.T., Holder, E., Lachs, M., O'Brien, J.G., & Sanders, A.B. (1993). Diagnostic and treatment guidelines on elder abuse and neglect. *Archives of Family Medicine, 2,* 371-388.

Bass, D.M., Anetzberger, G.J., Ejaz, F.K., & Nagpaul, K. (2000). Screening tools and referral protocol for stopping abuse against older Ohioans: A guide for service providers. *Journal of Elder Abuse & Neglect, 13* (2), 23-38.

Baumhover, L.A., Beall, S.C., & Pieroni, R.E. (1990). Elder abuse: An overview of social and medical indicators. *Journal of Health and Human Resource Administration, 12* (4), 414-433.

Blakely, B.E., & Dolon, R. (1991). The relative contributions of occupation groups in the discovery and treatment of elder abuse and neglect. *Journal of Gerontological Social Work, 17* (1/2), 183-199.

Brandl, B. (2000). Power and control: Understanding domestic violence in later life. *Generations, 24* (11), 39-45.

Brandl, B., & Raymond, J. (1997). Unrecognized elder abuse victims: Older abused women. *Journal of Case Management, 6* (2), 62-68.

Breckman, R.S., & Aldeman, R.D. (1988). *Strategies for helping victims of elder mistreatment.* Newbury Park, CA: Sage.

Collins, M. (1982). *Improving protective services for older Americans: A national guide series: Social worker role.* Portland, ME: University of Southern Maine, Center for Research and Advanced Study.

Daiches, S. (1983). *Protective services risk assessment: A new approach to screening adult clients.* New York: Project Focus.

Duke, J. (1993). *A national study of involuntary protective services to adult protective services clients.* Richmond, VA: National Association of Adult Protective Services Administrators and Virginia Department of Social Services.

Ferguson, D., & Beck, C. (1983). H.A.L.F.–A tool to assess elder abuse within the family. *Geriatric Nursing, 4,* 301-304.

Fulmer, T., & Anetzberger, G.J. (1995). *Knowledge about family violence interventions in the field of elder abuse.* Unpublished paper for the Committee on the Assessment of Family Violence Interventions of the National Research Council and Institute of Medicine.

Fulmer, T.T., & Gould, E.S. (1996). Assessing neglect. In L.A. Baumhover & S.C. Beall (Eds.), *Abuse, neglect, and exploitation of older persons: Strategies for assessment and intervention* (pp. 89-103). Baltimore: Health Professions Press.

Fulmer, T.T., & O'Malley, T.A. (1987). *Inadequate care of the elderly: A health care perspective on abuse and neglect.* New York: Springer Publishing Company.

Goodrich, C.S. (1997). Results of a national survey of state protective services programs: Assessing risk and defining victim outcomes. *Journal of Elder Abuse & Neglect, 9* (1), 69-86.

Gray-Vickrey, P. (2000). Protecting the older adult. *Nursing 2000, 30* (7), 34-38.

Heisler, C.J. (1991). The role of the criminal justice system in elder abuse cases. *Journal of Elder Abuse & Neglect, 3* (1), 5-34.

Hirsch, C.H., Stratton, S., & Loewy, R. (1991). The primary care of elder mistreatment. *Western Journal of Medicine, 170,* 353-358.

Hooyman, N.R. (1982). Mobilizing social networks to prevent elder abuse. *Physical & Occupational Therapy in Geriatrics, 2* (2), 21-35.

Jackson, R. (1999). Abuse and neglect in long-term care: A litigation boom threatens the industry. *Health Care Food & Nutrition Focus, 15* (6), 1, 3-5.

Johnson, T.F. (1991). *Elder mistreatment: Deciding who is at risk.* New York: Greenwood Press.

Jones, J., Dougherty, J., Schelble, D., & Cunningham, W. (1988). Emergency department protocol for the diagnosis and evaluation of geriatric abuse. *Annals of Emergency Medicine, 17,* 1006-1015.

Lachs, M.S., & Pillemer, K. (1995). Abuse and neglect of elderly persons. *The New England Journal of Medicine, 332* (7), 437-443.

Marshall, C.E., Benton, D., & Brazier, J.M. (2000). Elder abuse: Using clinical tools to identify clues of mistreatment. *Geriatrics, 55* (2), 42-53.

Miller, T.W., & Veltkamp, L.J. (1998). *Clinical handbook of adult exploitation and abuse.* Madison, CT: International Universities Press.

Moskowitz, S. (1998). Saving granny from the wolf: Elder abuse and neglect–The legal framework. *Connecticut Law Review, 31,* 77-204.

Nahmiash, D., & Reis, M. (2000). Most successful intervention strategies for abused older adults. *Journal of Elder Abuse & Neglect, 12* (3/4), 53-70.

National Research Council (2003). Elder mistreatment: Abuse, neglect, and exploitation in an aging America. Washington, DC: The National Academies Press.

Neale, A.V., Hwalek, M.A., Goodrich, C.S., & Quinn, K.M. (1997). Reason for case closure among substantiated reports of elder abuse. *The Journal of Applied Gerontology, 16* (4), 442-458.

Neale, A.V., Hwalek, M.A., Scott, R.O., Sengstock, M.C., & Stahl, C. (1991). Validation of the Hwalek-Sengstock elder abuse screening test. *The Journal of Applied Gerontology, 10* (4), 406-418.

Nerenberg, L. (2000). Developing a service response to elder abuse. *Generations, 24* (11), 86-92.

Ohio Department of Job and Family Services. (2003). *Adult protective services fact sheet for SFY 2003.* Columbus, OH: Author.

Payne, B.K. (2000). *Crime and elder abuse: An integrated perspective.* Springfield: IL: Charles C Thomas.

Phillips, L.R. (1983). Elder abuse–What is it? Who says so? *Geriatric Nursing, 4* (3) 167-170.

Phillips, L.R. (1988). The fit of elder abuse with the family violence paradigm, and the implications of a paradigm shift for clinical practice. *Public Health Nursing, 5* (4), 222-229.

Phillips, L.R., & Rempusheski, V.F. (1986). Making decisions about elder abuse. *Social Casework: The Journal of Contemporary Social Work, 67* (3), 131-140.

Podnieks, E. (1985). Elder abuse: It's time we did something about it. *The Canadian Nurse, 81* (11).

Polisky, R.A. (1995). Criminalizing physical and emotional elder abuse. *The Elder Law Journal, 3* (2), 377-411.

Quinn, M.J. & Tomita, S.K. (1997). *Elder abuse and neglect: Causes, diagnosis, and intervention strategies* (2nd ed.). New York: Springer Publishing Company.

Rathbone-McCuan, E., Travis, A. & Volyes, B. (1983). Family intervention: The task-centered approach. In J.I. Kosberg (Ed.), *Abuse and maltreatment of the elderly: Causes and interventions* (pp. 355-375). Littleton, MA: John Wright, PSG.

Reis, M., & Nahmiash, D. (1998). Validation of the Indicators of Abuse (IOA) screen. *The Gerontologist, 38*(4), 471-480.

Rosenblatt, D.E. (1996). Documentation. In L.A. Baumhover & S.C. Beall (Eds.), *Abuse, neglect, and exploitation of older persons: Strategies for assessment and intervention* (pp. 145-161). Baltimore: Health Professions Press.

Segal, S.R., & Iris, M.A. (1989). Strategies for service provision: The use of legal interventions in a systems approach to casework. In R. Filinson & S.R. Ingman (Eds.), *Elder abuse: Practice and policy* (pp. 104-116). New York: Human Sciences Press.

Sengstock, M.C., Hwalek, M., & Moshier, S. (1986). A comprehensive index for assessing abuse and neglect of the elderly. In Galbraith, M.W. (Ed.), *Elder abuse: Perspectives on an emerging crisis* (pp. 41-64). Kansas City, KS: Mid-America on Aging.

Sengstock, M.C., Hwalek, M., & Petrone, S. (1989). Services for aged abuse victims: Service types and related factors. *Journal of Elder Abuse & Neglect, 1* (4), 37-56.

Silverman, J., & Hudson, M.F. (2000). Elder mistreatment: A guide for medical professionals. *North Carolina Medical Journal, 61*(5), 291-296.

Simmelink, K. (1996). Lessons learned from three elderly sexual assault survivors. *Journal of Emergency Nursing, 22*(6), 619-621.

Stiegel, L. (1995), *Recommended guidelines for state courts handling cases involving elder abuse.* Washington, DC: American Bar Association Commission on Legal Problems of the Elderly.

Tatara, T. (1995). *An analysis of state laws addressing elder abuse, neglect, and exploitation.* Washington, DC: National Center on Elder Abuse.

Teaster, P. B. (2003). A response to the abuse of vulnerable adults: The 2000 survey of state adult protective services. Washington, DC: National Center on Elder Abuse.

Tomita, S.K. (1982). Detection and treatment of elderly abuse and neglect: A protocol for health care professionals. *Physical & Occupational Therapy in Geriatrics, 2* (2), 37-51.

Villmoare, E., & Bergman, J. (Eds.). (1981, February). *Elder abuse and neglect: A guide for practitioners and policy makers.* San Francisco: National Paralegal Institute.

Vinton, L. (1991). An exploratory study of self-neglectful elderly. *Journal of Gerontological Social Work, 18* (1/2), 55-67.

Vinton, L. (1992). Services planned in abusive elder care situations. *Journal of Elder Abuse & Neglect, 4* (3), 85-99.

Wilber, K.H., & Nielsen, E.K. (2002). Elder abuse: New approaches to an age-old problem. *The Public Policy and Aging Report, 12* (2), 1, 24-27.

Wolf, R. (2002). Risk assessment instruments. *National Center Elder Abuse Newsletter, 3* (1).

Wolf, R.S. (2000b). Elders as victims of crime, abuse, neglect, and exploitation. In M.B. Rothman, B.D. Dunlop, & P. Entzel (Eds.), *Elders, crime, and the criminal justice system: Myth, perceptions, and reality in the 21st century* (pp.19-42). New York: Springer Publishing Company.

Elder Abuse:
Case Studies for Clinical Management

Georgia J. Anetzberger, PhD, ACSW, LISW

SUMMARY. Elder abuse is best portrayed through the circumstances and viewpoints of its most involved parties–the victims and perpetrators of this problem. Three case studies provide a glimpse into elder abuse across rural and urban settings. Collectively they depict multiple abuse forms and consequences as well as differing family and cultural dynamics. *[Article copies available for a fee from The Haworth Document Delivery Service: 1-800-HAWORTH. E-mail address: <docdelivery@haworthpress.com> Website: <http://www.HaworthPress.com> © 2005 by The Haworth Press, Inc. All rights reserved.]*

KEYWORDS. Elder abuse case studies, self-neglect, domestic violence in later life, neglect, exploitation

For the purposes of this publication, clinical management of elder abuse will be considered through three case studies during two phases and involving four professional disciplines. Each of the case studies is a composite of several actual elder abuse situations, although names and identifying characteristics were changed to protect the anonymity of the victims and their family members. Most of these elder abuse situations were encountered by me, functioning as a clinician, administrator, or re-

---

Georgia J. Anetzberger is Research Associate, Visiting Nurse Association, Healthcare Partners of Ohio, Cleveland, Ohio.

[Haworth co-indexing entry note]: "Elder Abuse: Case Studies for Clinical Management." Anetzberger, Georgia J. Co-published simultaneously in *Clinical Gerontologist* (The Haworth Press, Inc.) Vol. 28, No. 1/2, 2005, pp. 43-53; and: *The Clinical Management of Elder Abuse* (ed: Georgia J. Anetzberger) The Haworth Press, Inc., 2005, pp. 43-53. Single or multiple copies of this article are available for a fee from The Haworth Document Delivery Service [1-800-HAWORTH, 9:00 a.m. - 5:00 p.m. (EST). E-mail address: docdelivery@haworthpress.com].

Digital Object Identifier: 10.1300/J018v28n01_03

searcher in the field of elder abuse. However, a few situations reflect elder abuse experienced by persons I know as relatives, friends, neighbors, or work associates. This is important. It underscores the fact that elder abuse is not just a problem for those we call clients, patients, service consumers, or research subjects. It is pervasive in American society and can be found among personal relations as well.

The case studies are written as short stories, because elder abuse situations represent personal accounts, best understood and approached on their own terms. As such, they reflect the immediate circumstances of victims and perpetrators as well as the complex array of individual characteristics, life histories, choices, problems, and social relations revealed through the nature of the elder abuse, and the meaning and response to it.

The three case studies illustrate diverse community settings, elder abuse forms, victim and perpetrator relations, and cultural backgrounds. With only three, there are obvious limitations to the amount of diversity represented. Nonetheless, among them both rural and urban communities are evident. Several elder abuse forms are presented, including self-neglect, physical and psychological abuse, neglect, and financial abuse. The case studies also portray a person living alone, a couple married for decades, and an adult child caring for her elderly parent. Finally, the lifestyles and cultures of persons who are lesbian or African American are depicted.

Each case study captures a moment in time, although some earlier history or background information is provided. Each also ends at a point of possible clinical intervention. However, by and large the specific nature and course of that intervention is neither obvious nor easily decided. Equally discomforting, the situations do not suggest simple solutions. Rather they leave the reader, and clinician, with a certain amount of dread that problem resolution will be at least challenging and at worst elusive and incomplete. These unsettling qualities are endemic among elder abuse situations.

The case studies are clinically examined in two phases. The first phase involves a discipline-specific role and perspective by an attorney, physician, nurse, or social worker. Each professional received the questions listed in Figure 1 and had the opportunity to consider them in case analysis and management. Each professional also was given substantial latitude in molding case specifics so that opportunities existed for elder abuse detection and clinical management. The second phase brings the four professionals together and undertakes clinical assessment and management as a multidisciplinary team. The importance of multi-disciplinary teams in elder abuse intervention is discussed later in this publication. This is followed by the team analysis of the three case studies presented here. It is hoped that together these descriptions offer understanding of major professional disciplines concerned with elder abuse identification, assessment, and intervention. In addition, the analyses seek to foster awareness about how the professional disciplines function both individually and collectively in clinical management of elder abuse situations.

JANE

Outside the wind is blowing off Lake Erie, threatening the rural county to the east of Cleveland with yet another blanket of "lake-effect snow." At last count five feet have accumulated. Any more and the state governor will declare emergency conditions.

Jane looks out of the only window in her home which can be easily accessed. The rest are hidden behind mounds of clutter–books and papers from her days as a high school history teacher, furniture and appliances from flea market sales and her parents' estate (dead more than fifty years), collected newspapers and clothing to sort and sell. The list of clutter and the reasons for its existence are many and varied, and mostly not relevant. The clutter is just there. "I'll get to it sometime," Jane thinks, but never does. It's too massive and overwhelming.

The snow starts and gives the appearance of continuing a long time. It covers Jane's mailbox across the road. Drifts submerge half of what used to be a barn near the house, now mostly fallen and rotting timber. The road is impassable. It will be days before any travels can be made on its icy and snow-covered surface.

For some, the isolation imposed by what the local newspaper labels "the worst winter in a decade" might be lonely and frightening. Jane isn't one of these people. She has nearly always managed on her own. "I like it that way. I certainly don't want other people around who think they can involve themselves in everybody's business."

Jane is 78-years-old and almost a life-long resident of the county. An only child of farmers, she decided to become a teacher because "I was smarter than the other kids, and liked to boss people." Education wasn't emphasized at home. Anyway, her parents couldn't afford for Jane to attend college, so she financed it herself. She completed both her bachelor's and master's degrees in succession by attending college in neighboring counties and working for local residents–as a farm laborer, housekeeper, whatever. She lived in her parents' home during this period. Af-

FIGURE 1. Questions to Consider in Analyzing the Three Elder Abuse and Neglect Case Studies

From the perspective of your particular professional discipline:

1. How are you likely to encounter this person? What reaction is the person likely to have to you?
2. What additional information do you need in order to proceed?
3. What questions will you ask in your initial interview with this person?
4. What elements will comprise your clinical assessment of the situation?
5. What clinical findings (e.g., signs and risk factors of abuse or neglect) will you look for? How will you document them?
6. What tools or protocols will you use in assessment and clinical management?
7. With whom will you consult in assessing the situation?
8. What do you see as the presenting problems in this case?
9. What is the level of risk or danger in the situation?
10. What are the goals in addressing this situation? Short-term? Long-term? What goals have greater priority?
11. What decision-making process will you employ in clinical management? Will certain principles or standards guide this process? What principles or standards?
12. What issues are you likely to encounter in assessment and intervention?
13. Are there ethical dilemmas?
14. What interventions are you likely to initiate? Immediately? Later?
15. To whom will you refer the client for assistance?
16. What professional or legal obligations do you have in this situation?
17. What do you see as your role and responsibility? In clinical management of this case?
18. How will you measure the impact of intervention and potential outcomes?
19. What is the likely prognosis for the client?
20. Under what circumstances will you close the case?

ter graduation she got a job with the Cleveland public school system, taking a small apartment a few blocks from where she taught.

Although never one to make friends willingly (some call her "aloof," others say "she thinks she's better than the rest of us"), Jane became attracted to a fellow teacher. The two women eventually decided to live together, returning to Jane's home county and buying a house on thirty acres of land. Commuting a distance of 45 miles might be time-consuming, but it provided the level of privacy that living near work never would.

For nearly a quarter century life for the two women had a certain routine. It was simple and pleasant, and it didn't involve much of anyone else after Jane's parents died, which happened a few years into the couple's relationship. Daily tasks surrounded teaching and maintaining a garden and several chickens and goats. The couple's main diversions were flea markets. There was always another item to buy and bring home to store. And, of course, there were their cats, an ever growing number and assortment of strays that found their way to the women's property and a new home.

When her partner died suddenly and unexpectedly from complications following surgery, Jane became severely depressed, even further withdrawn, angry at the world, and bitter about her circumstances. Only the cats and home routine seemed to sustain her.

Shortly after her partner's death, Jane had the opportunity to leave teaching with a pension for thirty years of service. She took it and left. The break was immediate and complete. Jane never returned, not even for a visit. She never contacted any of the school's teachers or staff with whom she shared space so many years, and they never contacted her. The few communications initiated by former students were never answered. Eventually, they stopped calling and writing as well.

The pain of her partner's death didn't subside as long as Jane was sober. Alcohol helped to make life bearable when nothing else did. In a sense, it represented a "loyal old friend." During college, Jane frequented the gay bars in Cleveland and Akron. It was part of lesbian culture and identity during the 1940s. Everyone was very closeted then. Those in public service occupations, like Jane, had to be especially careful about employers discovering their sexual orientation. Jobs could be lost, as well as housing and even freedom (jail wasn't out of the question).

Jane left the bars behind when she met her partner. However, drinking remained something she did, perhaps not a lot, but certainly daily. Now she drank a lot every day.

The snow continues to fall and the temperature drops. The only source of heat for the entire house is a fireplace located in the living room. Jane feeds it wood that she cut from fallen trees on her land last summer, but it's still cold and it hurts to lift the heavy logs. The furnace hasn't operated since 1992. Electricity is used for lights and cooking, but not for heat. Jane wanders around the house clothed in many layers of shirts and sweaters and pants. Her feet are warmed by woolen socks and papers stuffed in extra-sized boots. There's a thick woolen hat on her head, and lined leather work gloves on her hands. Jane hasn't changed any of them for weeks–it's too cold, not necessary, and why bother, she believes.

The sparks dance from the fire-place. Mostly they land on surrounding stone. Once in a while, however, they leap onto a mound of clutter.

Usually Jane manages to crush out these stray sparks before they cause any damage. Lately, she's missing more, because her eyesight is failing, or she's not getting there on time, because her arthritis is more disabling. The worst mishap resulted in a fire that destroyed a chair before it was extinguished. Jane burned her hands in the process. The local urgent care center physician dressed the wounds, and a visiting nurse stopped by the house to change the dressings, since Jane was unable to do this herself. That was almost a year ago. The charred chair remains where it was, a memorial to Jane's determination to manage on her own.

Besides the visiting nurse and Jane herself, no one has entered the house in twenty years. Neighbors learned long ago to "keep to themselves." They consider the house and land "eye sores," but few people are around to see them. Jane's only living relative is a distant cousin in Michigan, whose last contact resulted in an argument that made further contact unlikely. The number of cats has increased. There are perhaps thirty now. Jane is uncertain exactly how many, since some are inside cats and others are barn cats, and the barn cats come and go, often returning in the company of more, who stay.

Were it not for the snow, Jane might be going to town today. She does this monthly to buy groceries and other supplies. The trip will have to wait until better weather, but little food remains.

Driving used to be easier before Jane's eyesight changed. Now it's hard to see details, and impossible to navigate at night. But what makes driving really hard is the prospect of getting lost. Until a nearby intersection was closed and traffic diverted, it wasn't too much of a problem. Now the route seems unfamiliar, even confusing at times. Recently it took a couple hours to make the usual thirty minute trip to town.

Other things also have bothered Jane recently. She watches a cardinal land on a nearby tree. Its color is in great contrast with the snow. Jane tries to remember if she had breakfast this morning, and can't. "It doesn't really matter, I suppose" she reasons.

WANDA AND CARL

"Wanda," calls Carl from the upstairs bedroom. It's the seventh time he's tried to get her attention in the past half-hour. Wanda doesn't respond. It's not that she hasn't heard her husband of nearly fifty years. It's just that, "I don't give a damn what he wants. He oughta just shut up and leave me alone." Wanda watches her favorite soap opera as she folds just-laundered clothing. She closes her mind to Carl's calls. Long ago she shut down any feeling for him as well.

At age 68 Carl is dying of cancer. Once a large and robust man, he now is frail and weak. His hollowed cheeks and sunken eyes bear little resemblance to those of the ex-Marine, who served in the Korean War, and former businessman, whose job it was to turn around unprofitable paper supply distributors. That frequently meant cutting benefits, firing personnel, even closing certain operations. Carl was nicknamed "The Terminator." From management above him, it represented a compliment. "Carl will do whatever it takes to turn a profit." From employees at distribution centers under his authority, it represented a recrimination, or worse.

Carl applied the qualities that made him successful as a Marine and businessman to his personal life. A concept of himself as "head of the household" meant that his wife and son were expected to take his direction in all matters. This led Wanda to feel like a failure, because she never did things quite as well or as fast as Carl wanted. Wanda's perceived shortcomings were met by verbal condemnations from Carl that began shortly after their marriage vows and seemed to intensify with time. They became acute during periods when profit margins at Carl's work remained small and he was under both personal and company pressure to increase them.

Sometimes words became actions, as Carl's anger exploded into a shower of slamming fists, thrown books, and smashed dishes. In these moments Wanda and their son became silent, in part frozen in fear, in part waiting for the tirade to pass. Usually it did fairly quickly, only to return the next time things didn't quite go as expected.

Three times Carl's anger was physically directed at Wanda. The first occasion was ignited when Wanda and Carl entertained Carl's boss in their home. Carl interpreted one of Wanda's remarks as a public criticism against him. Later that evening they argued and he took a shoe and beat her so hard that she went to the hospital emergency department for stitches. On another occasion Wanda spilled coffee on the dining room rug right before some of Carl's work associates were to arrive. With one great heave, Carl threw Wanda against the wall. No bones broke, but Wanda's left arm and shoulder were a mass of bruises. The most recent occasion happened a few years ago, just after Carl retired from work at age 62. In a sense, Wanda became the only person that Carl could "boss" in the absence of employees. That made things even harder for Wanda. One day she didn't immediately clean up a spill that occurred while cooking Carl's lunch. When Carl slipped on it, his anger poured out in the form of boiling water thrown at the spill and splashing Wanda on both legs. Her burns were treated at the hospital emergency department. When the attending physician asked about the origins of the burns, Wanda attributed them to "clumsiness" on her part.

Still, Wanda never left Carl. Sometimes she wondered if she could bear living even one more minute in the face of his relentless demands and complaints, but she stayed. Carl's most frequent comments to Wanda were, "You're so stupid! Don't you know how to do anything right?!" and "This place is a mess! What have you been doing all day?!" Both Catholics, divorce seemed out of the question. Anyway, where was Wanda to go, what was she to do, and how was she to manage without Carl?

Wanda and Carl married in 1953, when she was 17 and he was 19. Wanda dropped out of high school to be with Carl, home on leave from the Marines. She hadn't known Carl very long. They met at a dance, and then he shipped out for combat. Most of their contact afterwards, until they married a year later, took place via the mail.

Throughout the marriage, Wanda remained a homemaker and mother. "I wasn't trained for anything, and Carl thought a 'woman's place is in the home.'" Their first two children were stillborn. Their son arrived during year five of the marriage. He was a joy to Wanda and a discipline challenge for Carl. The son left home at 18, moved to a distant state, and rarely comes back to visit.

At first, marrying Carl seemed like the right move for Wanda. She wanted to get away from her abusive father. She wasn't quite sure what to do with her life, and being Carl's wife seemed like the best option available. Anyway, "Carl was as handsome as they get in his uniform. He was smart, already had a year of college, and knew he was going to make something of himself. He had these great ambitions, and I wanted to go along."

Carl's job meant that the family never stayed long in any locale. Within the first half of their marriage, Carl and Wanda moved a dozen times. As a result, Wanda had few friends. Because of her lack of education, she felt that she had little in common with the wives of Carl's work associates. Because she saw herself as lacking any special talents or skills, Wanda never joined clubs or volunteered her time. Companionship, such as it was, rested with Carl and their son, until the son left, and then there was only Carl–strong, opinionated, argumentative Carl.

Carl tries to move in the bed. It's hard even to shift to another side, nearly impossible to turn over. In his fifties Carl developed diabetes. It became uncontrollable, and both legs were amputated below the knees two years ago. Then he was diagnosed with terminal cancer. Weakness and pain are constants. There is little he can do on his own. "I'm so thirsty," admits Carl. "Where's Wanda?"

Wanda slowly climbs the stairs and enters the bedroom where Carl is lying. "Carl, can't you see I'm busy?! What do you want now?" Wanda puts a glass half filled with water just beyond easy grasp for Carl, then roughly turns him onto his other side. "Don't think I'm at your beck and call. You know, you could do a lot more for yourself if you tried. You're no baby."

With that last remark, Wanda closes the bedroom door and leaves. Downstairs she goes through the stack of medical bills that have accumulated during Carl's illnesses. "He's using up all our savings," she mutters to herself and decides that a little less care won't make a whole lot of difference to someone who is dying anyway. Acting on that thought, Wanda telephones Carl's physician and announces, "Carl has decided that enough's enough. I won't be bringing him in anymore. This isn't working, and Carl's not getting any better."

BRENDA AND HARRIET

Brenda sits at the kitchen table, eating a breakfast that mainly consists of coffee and leftovers from yesterday's supper. Her eldest daughter put it together from yet other leftovers–a unique combination of pork, rice, potatoes, and onions. "Not bad," assesses Brenda, as she struggles to wake up from her evening shift as nursing assistant for a nearby nursing home. Unfortunately, her relief called in sick again, so a shift that ordinarily concludes at 11:00 pm stretched until morning instead.

It is nearly noon. Technically the food being eaten is probably more lunch than breakfast. Whatever might be the name, it satisfies Brenda, who lingers at the table long after every morsel is consumed, staring into space, sipping a second cup of strong coffee. Brenda is tired, physically, emotionally, and spiritually, from work that strains the back and impales the soul. The tasks seem unending that must be performed on behalf of the 14 residents on her unit–dressing, bathing, feeding, toileting– and that's just some of it. "When it's done, it isn't. You just start over again," acknowledges Brenda to no one in particular.

For this Brenda receives nine dollars an hour. The administrator is careful that none of the assistants achieves full-time work status. As a result, Brenda has no health insurance or other benefits, and she usually works at one or two additional homes to supplement her income.

Recently separated from the father of her children, Brenda lives with them and her mother in her mother's home. Harriet is nearly 70, with numerous chronic illnesses from diabetes to hypertension. In Brenda's opinion, however, the worst of them is Alzheimer's disease. Brenda is able to handle Harriet's medications and make sure that her daily needs are met. Much harder is dealing with the behaviors that result from Harriet's progressive dementia.

Brenda and Harriet were close while Brenda was growing up. Harriet worked as a domestic for several families from the affluent eastern suburbs. Every day she took one, two, even three buses to the homes of the white families that employed her, and every evening she returned to the city and the house where Brenda and her brothers were raised and where Brenda and her children have returned to live. Brenda had a happy childhood–lots of work, but also lots of love. She never met her father. He died in prison, killed by another inmate during a fight. Harriet described him as a "good man, but not one you could count on for much."

Brenda spent her twenties and early thirties living on her own. It was never easy, but she survived, even as a single mother with two young daughters. Initially she tried to support herself as a domestic, like her mother. But she hated cleaning other people's homes. A friend took training to become a nursing assistant, so Brenda did as well. She liked the work and the pay was better. However, she had trouble finding the right place to be employed. In the last five years she had jobs at six different nursing homes. Things always start out fine, then something happens–she is late "once too often" ("Don't they understand I have kids who get sick?!"), or a resident complains that Brenda slapped her ("She's always accusing people of doing something to her. The way she acts, it's more surprising if they don't."), or she doesn't like the charge nurse ("Who does she think she is telling me what to do!")–and she leaves. In a big city, there is always another nursing home to accept your job application, so finding alternative work is never very hard.

Hard is working with demented residents all evening and then coming home to a demented mother. For Brenda, being around Harriet is worse than being around a hundred demented residents. Harriet wanders at night, so it's impossible for Brenda to sleep when she returns home. Harriet is anxious and suspicious. She paces the house, can rarely sit still. She accuses Brenda's daughters, ages 8 and 6, charged with watching her in Brenda's absence, of theft of anything she can't find. When Brenda's around, Harriet follows her, talking, saying the same things over and over again. "She's gonna drive me mad," decides Brenda.

Placing Harriet in a nursing home would make things less stressful for Brenda. But then Harriet's house would need to be sold, and where would Brenda and her daughters live? Anyway, Harriet has been adamant, "I don't want to be anywhere other than here when I die. I certainly don't want to be in one of those homes for old folks." Other sources of help, like adult day care, might require Harriet to use the little savings that she managed to accumulate during her many years of hard work. Brenda doesn't want other people to have savings that "rightfully" belong to her and her daughters. "Money should stay in the family," she reasons. "Anyway, we're earning it, taking care of Mama like we are."

Brenda continues to stare into space as Harriet turns the corner and enters the kitchen. "Where's my purse? Did you take it?" asks Harriet.

Brenda looks up, swallows hard, wants to run, but stays anchored to her chair. Her oldest daughter had taken Harriet's purse and spent the money in it on dolls and games. It wasn't the first time that this had happened. Brenda sighs, because it probably won't be the last time either. Her reply, however, does not reveal her thoughts. "No, Mama, I didn't take your purse. You probably just misplaced it."

"No, I didn't. You know where it is. You're just not telling me." The dialogue continues until Brenda can stand it no longer. "If you don't stop, Mama, I'm gonna place you in one of those old folks' homes you can't stand. How would you like that?!" Harriet is silenced for a minute, and Brenda takes the opportunity to leave. "I'm going to the store, Mama. I'll be back later."

When Brenda returns three hours later, Harriet is gone. A call from the emergency department of the local hospital reveals that Harriet was found at a shopping area nearly a mile from the house, looking for Brenda. The police brought Harriet to the emergency department for evaluation. After Harriet returns home via ambulance, Brenda yells at her, "Can't you just stay put for a little while?! You'll get me in trouble. Now I'm going to have to lock you in your room whenever I'm gone. It's your fault that it has to be this way."

Following her outburst Brenda sits down and cries. It feels like her tears will fall indefinitely. Harriet no longer seems like the mother who raised Brenda. For that matter, Brenda doesn't seem like herself either. Unexpectedly Harriet puts her hand on Brenda's shoulder. For the briefest of moments, her mother has returned.

Elder Abuse:
The Attorney's Perspective

Maria Schimer, JD, MPH, RN

SUMMARY. Three cases have been presented for multidisciplinary consideration. This article analyzes them from the prospective of a practicing attorney. As such, it begins with a discussion of the ethical principles that govern legal practice, specifically in the area of elder law. The discussion which follows examines key points of law pertaining to elder abuse, neglect, and exploitation including key definitions; the duty of the attorney to report suspected cases; and rights of and procedural safeguards afforded to the alleged victim in a court proceeding to involuntarily enforce a protective order. The issue of guardianship also is briefly explored, as well as the requirements for involuntary confinement in a mental health facility. A consideration of how an attorney might become involved in each case and the underlying assumptions precedes an analysis of the cases set forth earlier. The final section summarizes key points of the article. *[Article copies available for a fee from The Haworth Document Delivery Service: 1-800-HAWORTH. E-mail address: <docdelivery@haworthpress. com>Website: <http://www.HaworthPress.com> © 2005 by The Haworth Press, Inc. All rights reserved.]*

KEYWORDS. Elder law, role of attorney, protective services law, guardianship, civil commitment

---

Maria Schimer is affiliated with the Office of Geriatric Medicine and Gerontology, Northeastern Ohio Universities College of Medicine, Rootstown, Ohio.

[Haworth co-indexing entry note]: "Elder Abuse: The Attorney's Perspective." Schimer, Maria. Co-published simultaneously in *Clinical Gerontologist* (The Haworth Press, Inc.) Vol. 28, No. 1/2, 2005, pp. 55-82; and: *The Clinical Management of Elder Abuse* (ed: Georgia J. Anetzberger) The Haworth Press, Inc., 2005, pp. 55-82. Single or multiple copies of this article are available for a fee from The Haworth Document Delivery Service [1-800-HAWORTH, 9:00 a.m. - 5:00 p.m. (EST). E-mail address: docdelivery@haworthpress.com].

http://www.haworthpress.com/web/CG
Digital Object Identifier: 10.1300/J018v28n01_04

WHO IS MY CLIENT?

The first question an attorney must answer before proceeding with any legal matter is "who is my client?" Is the client the person who walks in the door with a question, who pays the bill, or whose property or life is affected? The answer to these questions will immediately define for the attorney whose interests are paramount and what must be done to assure that those interests are promoted and protected.

Generally, a person who consults an attorney (1) possesses the requisite legal capacity to appreciate the nature and circumstances of the legal matters at hand; (2) is consulting the attorney about his/her own affairs; (3) will be signing an agreement of representation which sets forth the matters under consideration; and (4) will be paying the bill for services rendered from their own funds. However, when a family member or other person asks to be present during consultations and to "assist" in the conduct of matters that will affect the life or property of the older adult, important questions about the representation must be addressed. In some cases, admonitions about protecting the attorney-client privilege must be given; precautions must be observed; conditions of payment must be clarified; and, in some cases, representation must even be refused.

Older adults are particularly vulnerable to financial exploitation. The incidence of elder exploitation is increasing for several reasons including the national increase in the older adult population.[1] Almost one third of all older adults live alone.[2] The majority of these solitary seniors are women. Persons who live alone are more easily abused and exploited because their activities are not scrutinized regularly, and a solitary older adult has fewer opportunities to access and receive help from trustworthy advisors or advocates.[3] Additionally, older adults generally have significant financial resources including homes, cars, and bank accounts that make them attractive targets for the unscrupulous.[4]

When another person accompanies an older adult who is consulting an attorney, the attorney should speak to the older adult alone. The older adult should be questioned to ascertain the older adult's understanding of the legal matters under review; whether the proposed actions are being undertaken of the older adult's free will;[5,6] and whether the person accompanying them will benefit from the proposed actions or transactions. The attorney must endeavor to handle all consultations privately with the client to preserve attorney-client privilege.[7] A letter of representation should be drawn to define the scope of the representation, who will be billed and on what basis, and from whom payment will be accepted. An attorney must never accept compensation from anyone other than the client, except under very specific circumstances, and only after full disclosure. If an attorney accepted compensation from a third party, such actions could cause the attorney to run afoul of the ethical considerations set forth for practice of law in Ohio[8] and most other states.

If an attorney has reason to believe that the older adult is being exploited, he/she should counsel the older adult regarding this belief. If the older adult appears unable to act competently or independently, the attorney should refuse to accept employment. Certain other duties may arise under law and the ethical rules that govern the practice of law. These are discussed below.

ETHICAL CONSIDERATIONS

Ohio Code of Professional Responsibility

Lawyers in Ohio are required to follow, not only the letter and spirit of the law, but also the ethical principles established for the profession by the state Supreme Court. The situation is comparable in other states. The Supreme Court adopted the Code of Professional Responsibility (the Code) in 1970. It is organized into nine Canons, forty Disciplinary Rules (DR's), and one hundred and thirty-nine Ethical Consideration's (EC). The Canons state basic ethical precepts. They are mandatory in nature and embody the general concepts from which the EC's and DR's are derived.[9] The EC's "are aspirational in character and represent the objective toward which every member of the profession should strive."[10] The DR's are mandatory rules of conduct; they state "the minimum level of conduct below which no lawyer can fall without being subject to disciplinary action."[11]

The American Bar Association has adopted Model Rules which are not binding on attorneys in Ohio, but are instructive. They provide insight into issues not covered by the Code, and a national perspective on the ethical standards for the practice of law. The Code and the Model Rules are, not surprisingly, similar in many respects; however, they do differ on key points pertaining to the representation of persons with limited cognitive ability or insight into their legal matters.

The Preamble to the Model Rules describes the various functions of an attorney. These include: advisor, advocate, negotiator, intermediary, spokesperson, and evaluator. The most important roles, in the context of the previously described case studies, are the roles of advisor and advocate. As an advisor, an attorney "provides a client with an informed understanding of the client's legal rights and obligations and explains their practical implications."[12] As an advocate, an attorney "zealously asserts the client's position . . ."[13] However, the roles of intermediary, spokesperson, and evaluator become important in the ultimate resolution of any such matters. As an intermediary, the lawyer examines both sides of an issue and then seeks to reconcile the divergent interests. Finally, as an evaluator and spokesperson, the attorney examines the client's affairs and reports them as necessary to the client and where appropriate to others.

Preserving the Confidences and Secrets of the Client

Ohio's Canon 4 requires that an attorney "preserve the confidences and secrets of his client."[14] A "confidence" is limited to "information protected by the attorney-client privilege . . ." A "secret" is information gained in the professional relationship that the client "has requested be held inviolate or the disclosure of which would be embarrassing or would be likely to be detrimental to the client."[15] One of the EC that flows from this Canon instructs attorneys to preserve the confidences and secrets of their clients in order to encourage the client to disclose all the information necessary to assist the client in taking full advantage of the legal system. This obligation is even broader than the statutorily created evidentiary attorney-client privilege.

However, the EC's do not preclude a lawyer from revealing information under certain circumstances. These include situations in which the client consents after full disclosure, when it is necessary to perform professional employment, when a DR permits it, or when it is required by law.[16] In addition, DR 4-101 (C) provides, that a lawyer may reveal the confidences of a client "after full disclosure . . . when permitted by the Disciplinary Rules or required by law or court order." Finally, the rule allows disclosure if it is the "intention of his client to commit a crime and the information necessary to prevent the crime." Criminal offenses are defined by statute,[17] each of which must be narrowly and strictly construed.

What is the appropriate course of action if a client discloses to an attorney that he/she is "getting his/her affairs in order" because he/she is planning to commit suicide? In Ohio, suicide is not a crime. However, a 1980 New York case, *People v. Fentress*,[18] made a thoughtful and significant ruling when it stated "to exalt the oath of silence in the face of imminent death by suicide, would . . . be not only morally reprehensible, but ethically unsound." The American Bar Association, Commission on Ethics and Professional Responsibility, opined "the disclosure of a client's intention to commit suicide is ethical, even if suicide is not a crime in the jurisdiction."[19]

Zealous Representation

Ohio Canon 7 states, "A Lawyer Should Represent a Client Zealously Within the Bounds of the Law." The first EC under this Canon provides that it is the "duty of a lawyer . . . to represent his client zealously within the bounds of the law."[20] This EC notes that the members of the legal profession have the duty to assist members of the public to secure and protect all of their available legal rights and benefits, since each member of our society is entitled to have his conduct judged and regulated in accordance with the law, and to seek any lawful objective through all legally permissible means.[21]

The second EC under this notes that "the bounds of the law in a given case are often difficult to ascertain . . . limits and specific meaning of apparently relevant law may be made doubtful."[22] Any practicing attorney will be quick to note that cases may range from those that are well settled through clear statutes and common law standards to those fraught with conflicting authority and the absence of precedent. The third EC[23] is instructive in handling matters where the bounds of the law are uncertain. It provides that the actions of the lawyer may depend on whether he/she is serving as an advocate or advisor. While attorneys often serve as an advocate and advisor, the two roles are different. "[A]n advocate . . . deals with past conduct and must take the facts as he finds them." In this role the attorney must act zealously, construe all doubt in favor of the client, and, within the confines of truth and law, apply as positive an interpretation of the facts and governing law as is possible. By contrast, a lawyer serving as an advisor "primarily assists his client in determining the course of future conduct and relationships." When acting as an advisor, the attorney's duty is to advise the client about what the law in the area is likely to be.

The eleventh EC under this Canon notes that the "responsibilities of a lawyer may vary according to the intelligence, experience, mental condition or age of the client . . . or the nature of the proceeding."[24] Thus an attorney is required to assess the mental functioning and intelligence of a client during the course of representation. That requires the attorney to communicate in a manner that makes the legal considerations clear enough to the client that the client is able to make a meaningful decision based upon their goals, values, and individual circumstances. The EC places additional burdens on the attorney of a client who has any mental or physical condition that rendered him incapable of making a considered judgment on his/her own behalf. For example, if a client with a disability lacks a legal representative (e.g., guardian) and is faced with a court proceeding, the lawyer may be required to make decisions on behalf of the client.[25] More specifically, in the case where a lawyer represents a person of questionable mental capacity who is facing eviction, demolition of property, or criminal charges, the lawyer may have to enter pleas or make motions on behalf of the client that the client does not fully understand to protect the rights and interests of the client.

Further, the EC's require that if the client is "capable of understanding the matter . . . or of contributing to the advancement of his interests, regardless of whether he is disqualified from performing certain acts, the lawyer should obtain from him all possible aid."[26] This EC implies that even if a client is of limited ability, the lawyer should try to ascertain from the client how the client feels about the issues at hand, what options are available, and any other relevant information. Thus, even if a client is impaired in one area, the attorney should discern whether the client is able to understand information and meaningful choices in other areas.

If the disability of the client and the lack of a legal representative compel the lawyer to make decisions to safeguard the interests of the client, the lawyer must act with care to safeguard and advance the interests of his client. This places an enhanced fiduciary duty on the lawyer. Lawyers are always required to act with reasonable care to safeguard the interests of the client; under these particular circumstances, the lawyer must act with the utmost of care. However, such representation should not go on long term without the intervention of the Probate Court. Upon reviewing the matter, the Probate Court may appoint the lawyer as the person's guardian. This would place the actions of the attorney under the scrutiny of the Court that acts as the "super guardian" of persons who are incompetent.

The EC's also make it obvious that a lawyer "cannot perform any act or make any decision which the law requires his client to perform or make, either acting for himself if competent, or by a duly constituted representative if legally incompetent."[27] Therefore, if the clients clearly do not understand the nature and extent of their circumstances; cannot participate meaningfully in decisions regarding their interests; or cannot provide for themselves because of a mental disability, then, once again, the lawyer has the duty to assist in acquiring a legal representative to assist them.

Model Rule 1.14, Client's Under a Disability

Under the American Bar Association's Model Rules, an attorney is obligated to try to maintain the normal attorney-client relationship even when the "client's ability to make adequately considered decisions" is impaired by mental disability or other reason.[28] The comment on this Rule recognizes that although a client may have a disability, he/she often has "the ability to understand, deliberate upon, and reach conclusions about matters affecting the client's own well-being."[29]

This Rule further states that a lawyer may seek "the appointment of a guardian or take other protective actions . . . only when . . . the client cannot act in the client's own interest."[30] The comment on this Rule indicates that a lawyer must often act as a "de facto guardian." This, however, should not continue long term, because it puts the lawyer in the place of the client. It also presents opportunities for the unscrupulous attorney to take advantage of an incompetent client since the attorney would often have complete authority over the affairs of another with no oversight. The comment also suggests that the attorney may consult an appropriate diagnostician to ascertain whether a long-term guardian is necessary.

In 1996, the American Bar Association Standing Committee on Ethics and Professional Responsibility issued a formal Opinion in which it stated, "a lawyer may take appropriate action on behalf of a client with a disability." Under the Opinion, lawyers would be allowed to seek a guardian for a person the lawyer believed was confused and acting under the influence of another, "in order to protect the client and the attorney." Under this Opinion, a lawyer is also permitted to take appropriate steps to "gain insight into the client's capacity, and to undertake protection of the client's rights."

LEGAL CONSIDERATIONS

Is the Older Adult Competent?

Simply because an adult engages in eccentric or risky behavior does not make the person incompetent. Generally, persons over the age of 18 in the state of Ohio are considered competent to choose where, how, and with whom they will live; how they will use and dispose of property; and how they will establish and realize their life plans and goals. The Constitutions and the laws of the United States and Ohio guarantee these rights unless very important considerations override the exercise of personal autonomy.

The ethical principle of autonomy is rooted in the deontological tradition of Kant. This principle emphasizes respect for the person and holds that individuals should be allowed to establish and carry out their own life plans and goals so long as their actions do not infringe on the rights of others. Autonomy is understood to include a cluster of notions, including: self-determination, freedom, independence, and liberty of choice and action.[31] Autonomy, however, is predicated on several assumptions. These assumptions include that one is competent, free from duress (i.e., the action is voluntary) and that the decision is informed (i.e., there is understanding of the key issues involved and there is no fraud or deceit involved).[32]

Competence is a threshold legal issue that must be addressed before an attorney undertakes important actions or transactions on behalf of the client. The law is clear; a competent adult is accorded the freedom to make eccentric, risky, and even detrimental choices. The incompetent adult, by contrast, is not permitted to make, of his/her own accord, even reasonable and sensible choices.

The Ohio Revised Code (O.R.C.) defines as "incompetent" any person who is "so mentally impaired as a result of a mental or physical illness or disability, or mental retardation, or chronic substance abuse, that he is incapable of taking proper care of himself or his property . . . "[33] State laws vary in their specific provisions around the concept of incompetence, although elements found in Ohio law are not uncommon elsewhere. This standard establishes that a person who is so mentally impaired that he/she cannot function within and manage his/her environment could be a candidate for referral to the Probate Court for consideration of proper safeguards. Such safeguards might include the appointment of a guardian or conservator. Depending on the surrounding circumstances, the attorney may also have a duty to report the matter to the County Department of Job and Family Services (CDJFS) as discussed below.

The Code, as set forth above, would require the attorney representing a person reasonably believed to be incompetent to take immediate steps to safeguard the person's interests in any court proceeding. However, a careful and conscientious attorney should not assist an incompetent person to complete important transactions. If an attorney assists an incompetent person to complete such transactions as the execution of a Will, or the transfer of real estate, these transactions could be voided in the future by interested parties, and could result in limitations of the attorney's license or charges of malpractice.

Defining Adult Abuse, Neglect, and Financial Exploitation in Ohio

The Ohio Revised Code (O.R.C.) specifically defines adult abuse, neglect or exploitation. The term "adult" refers to a person that is at least 60 years of age and "who is handicapped by the infirmities of aging or who has a physical or mental impairment which prevents the person from providing for the person's own care or protection, and who resides in an independent living arrangement."[34] Persons between the ages of 18 and 60 do not have protections under the statute in Ohio. Persons who live in nursing homes receive protections under another statute.

Abuse is defined as the "the infliction upon an adult by self or others of injury, unreasonable confinement, intimidation, or cruel punishment with resulting physical harm, pain, or mental anguish."[35] Physical harm includes any "bodily pain, injury, impairment, or disease suffered by an adult."[36] Neglect is defined as " the failure of an adult to provide for self the goods or services necessary to avoid physical harm, mental anguish, or mental illness, or the failure of a caretaker to provide such goods or services."[37] Exploitation under the statute is "the unlawful or improper act of a caretaker using an adult or an adult's resources for monetary or personal benefit, profit, or gain."[38]

Non-Support Distinguished from Neglect

In 1974, the Ohio legislature consolidated many non-support features of Ohio law into O.R.C. §2919.21. This Section of the O.R.C. provides that no person "shall abandon, or fail to provide adequate support to . . . [t]he person's spouse, as required by law; . . . [t]he persons aged or infirm parent, . . . who from the lack of ability and means is unable to provide adequately for the parent's own support." The offense of non-support is separate from neglect and is considered a less serious offense. Generally, a person will be charged under this section, rather than the neglect section of the elder abuse law, when the person who is not supported is not at risk of "serious harm." A case emanating from the 9th District of Ohio, decided by the Ohio Supreme Court in 1998, makes clear that this statute "requires an adult child to provide adequate support for his or her dependent parent if the parent is in need of financial assistance and the adult child has the financial means to provide such support."[39] This case also provides that the support referred to is financial support and not support of any other kind, for example, emotional or caregiving support. Failure to provide financial support as provided for in the statute constitutes a misdemeanor of the first degree.[40]

An affirmative defense to the charge of non-support is that the person so accused "was unable to provide adequate support or the established support but did provide the support that was within the accused's ability and means."[41] Thus an adult child or spouse without the means to provide financial support to a dependent parent could assert that fact at a hearing on the issue. This defense, if supported by sufficient evidence, would prevent the spouse or child from legal culpability.

The Attorney's Duty to Report

The legislature in Ohio created a mandatory duty to report for many professionals. Under O.R.C. §5101.61 attorneys ostensibly have a mandatory duty to report any suspected elder abuse. Ohio is one of several states that, by statute, require attorneys to report abuse.[42] The statute does not provide for any consideration of how the lawyer comes to have knowledge of the alleged abuse, neglect, or exploitation. The author would argue that if the knowledge does not arise from the attorney-client relationship, the duty to report is clear and indisputable.

When the lawyer becomes aware of the situation in the context of the attorney-client relationship, an ethical conflict arises. The attorney is bound to protect the confidences and secrets of the client as outlined above. While the statute provides for an unqualified duty to report and thus provides a reason for the lawyer to breach the confidence of the client as outlined above, some legal experts would argue that the legislature overstepped its authority by establishing this duty. They would contend that the Ohio Constitution[43] gives the Supreme Court of Ohio the sole control over the conduct of attorneys and thus such a statute, created by the legislature, has no binding authority over the members of the legal profession.

The statute does provide protection against civil or criminal liability for any person who in good faith makes a report based upon the reasonable belief that abuse, neglect, or exploitation occurred.[44] However, the statute does not provide any protection from disciplinary action by the Supreme Court of Ohio. Since there is no case law on this specific point that would assist in resolving the issue, an attorney may feel conflicted on the matter.

O.R.C. §5101.61(A)(6)(g)(ii) states that "[a]ny attorney . . . having reasonable cause to believe that an adult is being abused, neglected, or exploited, or is in a condition which is the result of abuse, neglect, or exploitation shall immediately report such belief to the county department job and family services." Under the statute, an attorney who suspects abuse must immediately report such suspicions to the CDJFS.[45] The report may be made orally or in writing. The county department will, whenever possible, request the report in writing. All written reports made to the department should include the following:

1. The name, address, and approximate age of the adult who is the subject of the report;
2. The name and address of the individual responsible for the adult's care, if any individual is, and if the individual is known;
3. The nature and extent of the alleged abuse, neglect, or exploitation of the adult;
4. The basis of the reporter's belief that the adult has been abused, neglected, or exploited.[46]

If an attorney fails to report suspected abuse to the CDJFS, he or she may be fined up to five hundred dollars.[47]

"In Need of Protective Services"

Once a report of suspected abuse, neglect or exploitation is made, the CDJFS has a duty to investigate.[48] The investigation must be initiated within three working days or within twenty-four hours if an emergency exists. The investigation is required to include a "face-to-face visit with the adult . . . preferably in the adult's residence . . . and consultation with the person who made the report, if feasible, and agencies or persons who have information about the adult's alleged abuse, neglect, or exploitation."[49]

If during the course of an investigation of adult abuse, neglect or exploitation, any person "including the adult who is the subject of the investigation denies or obstructs access to the residence of the adult, the county . . . may file . . . a petition for a temporary restraining order to prevent interference or obstruction."[50] This restraining order is not issued lightly. The court issuing the order must make a finding that there is "reasonable cause to believe the person is being or has been abused, neglected or exploited and access . . . has been denied or obstructed."[51]

After obtaining the order from the court, the county investigator may be accompanied to the residence by a law enforcement officer. Upon completion of the investigation, the "department shall determine . . . whether or not the adult is in need of protective services."[52]

Protective services may be provided to any person who requests or consents to receive them only after an investigation is completed and a determination is made that there is a "need for protective services." If the person withdraws consent, the protective services are terminated.[53] If the county department determines that the adult is in need of protective services and is an "incapacitated person," the department may petition the court for an order to authorize the provision of protective services.[54]

"Incapacitated"

An incapacitated person is defined as a person who "is impaired for any reason to the extent that he lacks sufficient understanding or capacity to make and carry out reasonable decisions concerning his person or resources, with or without the assistance of a caretaker. Refusal to consent to the provision of services shall not be the sole determinative that the person is incapacitated. 'Reasonable decisions' are decisions made in daily living which facilitate the provision of food, clothing, and health care necessary for life support."[55] The reasonableness of the person's decisions will require consideration of the personal circumstances of the individual, as well as community standards for the basic necessities outlined above.

The petition to the court shall include the specific facts of the alleged abuse, neglect, or exploitation and shall include the service plan. The statute requires that a court hearing be held on the matter within fourteen days of the petition. The person who is the subject of the petition has full procedural due process rights including the "right to be present at the hearing, present evidence, and examine and cross-examine witnesses." Counsel shall represent the adult unless the right to counsel is "knowingly waived."[56] If the adult is indigent, "the court will appoint counsel . . . if the court determines that the adult lacks capacity to waive counsel, the court shall appoint counsel to represent the adult's interests."[57]

If the court finds by clear and convincing evidence four important factors, then the court will issue an order for protective services if they are locally available. The four factors that must be found include that the "adult has been abused, neglected, or exploited, is in need of protective services, and is incapacitated, and no person authorized by law or court order is available to give consent."[58] An initial order for protective services shall remain in effect for no longer than six months. Additional renewal orders may be applied for and issued for periods of no longer than one year.[59]

If the court orders a protective placement outside of the adult's normal place of residence, the court is bound to consider the "choice of residence of the adult." The court may order placement in a setting approved by the county department that must meet certain minimum requirements for safety, security, and requirements of daily living. However, the court "shall not order an institutional placement unless . . . no less restrictive alternative can be found to meet the needs of the individual."[60]

Guardianship

The EC's discussed in the sections above, make it clear that the attorney has an obligation to seek a legal representative for a client who the attorney believes lacks the legal capacity to act in his/her own interest.[61] In the short term, a lawyer must often act as a "de facto guardian." This, however, should not continue long term, because it puts the lawyer in the place of the client. It also presents opportunities for the unscrupulous attorney to take advantage of an incompetent client, since the attorney often would have complete, unfettered authority over the affairs of the client. Attorneys are allowed to seek a guardian for a person the lawyer believed was confused and acting under the influence of another to protect not only the client, but also the attorney in the situation.

Competency is at the heart of guardianship law.[62] In 1990, an estimated half million older adults in the United States were subject to guardianship.[63] A guardian is one appointed by the Probate Court to have "the care and management of the person of an incompetent."[64] The Court may appoint a guardian for an incompetent person "on its own motion or on application by an interested party" if the Court finds it to be "in the best interests" of the incompetent person to do so.[65] In Ohio, an incompetent person is one who is so *mentally impaired* "as a result of mental or physical illness or disability . . . that the person is incapable of taking proper care of the person's self or property . . . "[66]

Guardianship is usually a remedy of last resort since it deprives the adult of the rights of autonomy and self-determination. Because serious implications come into play with such determination, Ohio law builds in a number of important safeguards. Ohio is one of only two states (the other is California) that employs an investigator for guardianship proceedings.[67] The investigator serves several important functions: he/she "serves notice to the parties involved, informs the proposed wards of their rights, investigates the circumstances of the ward, and follows the guardianship after it is established."[68] The investigator must prepare a detailed report for the court describing the totality of the circumstances surrounding the petition for guardianship. The report must contain the following elements:

1. "a statement . . . that the notice was served and [that] . . . the alleged incompetent's rights to be present at the hearing, to contest any application for the appointment of a guardian for his person, estate or both, and to be represented by an attorney were communicated to him in a language or method of communication understandable to the alleged incompetent;
2. A brief description . . . of the physical and mental condition of the alleged incompetent;
3. A recommendation regarding the necessity for a guardianship or a less restrictive alternative;
4. A recommendation regarding the necessity of appointing . . . an attorney to represent the alleged incompetent."[69]

Prior to the appointment of a guardian, the court shall conduct a hearing. The report outlined above " . . . shall be made a part of the record in the case and shall be considered by the court prior to establishing any guardianship . . . "[70] At the hearing the alleged incompetent has the following procedural due process rights: "the right to be represented by independent counsel of his choice . . . to have friend or family member of his choice present . . . to have evidence of independent expert evaluation introduced . . . [if indigent] . . . to have counsel and independent evaluator appointed at court expense."[71]

The proposed guardian must appear at the hearing and prove by clear and convincing evidence that the person is incompetent. This requires the submission of sworn expert statements or testimony on the record. If there is evidence that a less restrictive alternative would protect the person, then the court will deny the guardianship in favor of the less restrictive alternative.

If appointed, the guardian has a duty to act in the person's best interests while faithfully and completely fulfilling the duties of a guardian as set forth in the statute.[72] In addition, the guardian must always obey the orders of the court because the court is the "superior guardian."[73]

Hospitalization of Mentally Ill Persons

Certain emergency circumstances may require that a person be confined involuntarily to a mental health facility. The O.R.C. provides that a "mentally ill person who is subject to hospitalization by court order" is a mentally ill person who "[r]epresents a substantial risk of physical harm to self as manifested by evidence of threats of, or attempts at, suicide or serious self-inflicted bodily harm . . . is unable to provide for and is not providing for the person's basic physical needs because of the person's mental illness . . . "[74] This section also provides that a person may be subject to hospitalization by court order if he/she "represents a substantial risk of physical harm to others . . . "[75] A person who is hospitalized under such circumstances has certain rights to him/herself from abuse of this power by the state. These rights include:

1. "Immediately make a reasonable number of telephone calls or use reasonable means to contact an attorney . . . to secure representation by counsel . . .
2. Retain counsel and have an independent expert evaluation . . . . if the person is unable to obtain an attorney or independent expert evaluation, be represented by court appointed counsel or have independent expert evaluation . . . at public expense."[76]

What About the Perpetrator?

Once the victim of abuse, neglect, or exploitation has been appropriately protected, the next issue becomes what to do with the perpetrator. Where the perpetrator is a family member, "any number of factors may precipitate abuse, including resentment, stress, substance abuse, a family history of violence, and the absence of care giving support."[77] The abuser may be "overwhelmed by the responsibility of caring for an infirm person, or of managing the financial burden of supporting a dependent elder."[78] These reasons do not excuse, but often do explain the behavior.

Chapter 29 of the O.R.C. defines the various criminal offenses in Ohio. These offenses range from minor misdemeanors that carry a penalty of not more than a one hundred dollar fine[79] to first-degree felonies that can carry the death penalty. The prosecuting attorney for the county in which the offense occurred has the discretion to determine the appropriateness of bringing charges based upon the totality of the circumstances involved.

While adult abuse, neglect, and exploitation may include a broad range of criminal offenses, some common offenses will be discussed briefly herein. Abuse encompasses "infliction upon an adult by self or others of injury, unreasonable confinement, or cruel punishment with resulting physical harm, pain, or mental anguish."[80] Such a definition could include Felonious Assault,[81] Domestic Violence,[82] and Aggravated Menacing.[83]

Neglect by the caregiver might easily come under O.R.C. §2903.16, "Failing to Provide for the Functionally Impaired." This statute provides that no caretaker "shall knowingly fail to provide a functionally impaired person under the caretaker's care with any treatment, care, goods, or service that is necessary to maintain the health or safety of the functionally impaired person when such failure results in physical harm." Violation of this section of the O.R.C. is a misdemeanor of the first degree. A misdemeanor of the first degree can result in no more than six months of imprisonment and no more than a thousand dollar fine.[84] If the caregiver recklessly, rather than knowingly, fails to provide for the functionally impaired person, the penalty is a misdemeanor of the second degree. This could result in imprisonment of up to ninety days and a fine of up to seven hundred and fifty dollars.[85]

The theft and fraud statutes within the O.R.C. easily encompass the criminal conduct involved in adult exploitation. For example, theft is defined in O.R.C. §2913.02. It states "No person, with purpose to deprive the owner of property or services, shall knowingly obtain or exert control over either the property or services in any of the following ways . . . without the consent of the owner or person to give consent . . . by deception . . . threat . . . intimidation." Whoever does so is guilty of theft. The level of the offense is measured in large part by the value of the property stolen, whether or not a firearm or dangerous ordnance was involved, and whether the victim is an "elderly or disabled adult." The level of the offense and the attendant criminal penalty is heightened if the victim is an older adult.

Another common theft offense under the O.R.C. is Misuse of Credit Cards.[86] Under the O.R.C., physical possession of the credit card is not required.[87] Unauthorized use of the card is all that is required. Forgery[88] is another frequent criminal offense that is encompassed under the definition of exploitation. If an unscrupulous person by some deception causes an older adult to sign a mortgage, Will, or other instrument which encumbers or conveys property or creates a pecuniary obligation on the part of the older adult, then the person could be charged with a violation of O.R.C. §2913.43, Secured Writings by Deception.

A victim of Domestic Violence or certain other offenses, including Aggravated Menacing, may file a motion with the court for Protective Orders.[89] The purpose of these Protective Orders is to ensure the safety and protection of the complainant and any other family or household members who might be at risk from the perpetrator. Unfortunately, no law enforcement authority can provide round-the-clock protection for the victim and the penalty for violation of such orders is only a misdemeanor of the first degree.

CASE ANALYSIS

How Would an Attorney Get Involved in These Cases?

Each of the cases discussed in the preceding article presents compelling social and ethical issues. However, it is unlikely that any of these cases would come to the attention of an attorney without some further trigger. The nature of the trigger will probably define the role and responsibilities of any attorney who would become involved.

Jane, based upon her profile, would not seek the assistance of an attorney so long as she is left alone. She has always been reclusive and would probably see no need for any services that an attorney might provide. In fact, most attorneys would argue that Jane should be left alone, even though her behavior is eccentric and risky, so long as she is able to appreciate the nature and extent of current circumstances and has not been adjudged incompetent by a court of law.

Jane might be appointed counsel under specific circumstances: if she were to be cited for a traffic violation of some magnitude (e.g., aggravated vehicular assault or homicide due to a drunk driving incident); if her rights were to be affected by the imposition of involuntary adult protective services; if the mental health authorities attempt to involuntarily confine her for more than 72 hours to a mental health facility, because she poses an imminent danger to herself or others (e.g., danger of fire); if she is facing a hearing to determine if she is incompetent to handle her affairs; or if her property were at risk, because she is violating some civil ordinance or public health standard. Without such a trigger, or the intervention of some other professional with a statutory duty to report her apparent self-neglect, she is likely to live out and end her life in this rural Ohio setting without ever coming to anyone but her nearest neighbor's attention.

Wanda and Carl present another familiar and compelling profile of the cycle of abuse where the line between victim and perpetrator shifts and is often obscured. They, like Jane, live behind closed doors. A significant trigger would be required for someone to open those doors and intervene. If Wanda's call to the physician declaring that Carl has decided that he has had enough did not ring true to the physician who has known them for some time, this might provide an entrée into their home and lives.

A physician who knew this family over time would probably want to have a discussion with Carl. The physician would want to ask Carl about his wishes regarding care. If he was unable to speak directly to Carl, he might ask Wanda about Carl's current pain level, mental status, ability to carry out activities of daily living, and the amount of burden Wanda is shouldering. The answers to these questions might provide the impetus for the physician to make a report to Adult Protective Services (APS) at the CDJFS. Such a report might cause the involvement of an attorney for both parties who clearly have different interests in this case.

Harriet, Brenda, and her children can live for a long time in relative obscurity in most large urban environments. From the outside, they might look like many families trying to "make things work" under difficult circumstances. Unless there was shouting or other apparent signs of violence, most neighbors would probably perceive Brenda as hard working, and sympathetic, because she is bearing a large burden of caring for an elderly mother and two small children. However, once the police bring Harriet into the Emergency Department at the local hospital, it is likely that the hospital social services personnel will contact APS at the CDJFS. Such a report will trigger an investigatory visit as outlined above. Other protective services agencies, such as Child Protective Services, may become involved after the initial APS visit as well. As with Wanda and Carl, Brenda and Harriet will likely require separate counsel because of the apparent conflict of interest under the facts of this case.

Jane

Jane is a reclusive woman, living in relative obscurity in a manner that has not changed much in over twenty years. She bothers no one and no one bothers her. The rural setting she chose to live in most of her adult life gives her the freedom to keep her house, property, and person in a manner of her own choosing. A more urban environment would constrain her significantly. In a city, housing and fire codes would have to be adhered to and public health and zoning ordinances could be enforced to require her to maintain her property within certain specified parameters. In a more urban setting a well-meaning neighbor or a concerned utility worker might call the APS to look in on Jane if they notice that she appears very cold, dazed, or otherwise in need.

In this case, there is some chance that the visiting nurse who saw Jane almost a year ago might phone APS to see if Jane was safe and warm during this especially bad winter. If the visiting nurse contacts APS, an investigation could be triggered as outlined above. Under the circumstances, it is likely that Jane will be found to be a self-neglecting individual who is in need of protective services within the meaning of the statute as outlined above. It is also likely that Jane would refuse to consent to voluntary protective services if that would impinge on her privacy and freedom to live her life as she sees fit. APS could not involuntarily provide protective services unless Jane is found to be, not only in need of such services, but also "incapacitated" by the court as outlined above.

If the attorney hired by Jane or appointed for her by the court believed that Jane was making knowing, albeit risky decisions, the attorney would have the duties of advocate and advisor as outlined above in the earlier section on zealous representation. To that end, the attorney advocate would seek to safeguard Jane's rights within the bounds of the law. The attorney would vigorously defend Jane's right to live as she chooses. The attorney would demonstrate that Jane knows the nature and extent of her circumstances, that she is able to make meaningful choices about her life style and that these choices are reasonable based upon some personal standard. The attorney would be required to assure that Jane received all the procedural protections provided for in the statute. She would, for example, through counsel be assured of the right to present evidence on her behalf and to question witnesses.

As an advisor, the attorney may well attempt to counsel Jane to cooperate voluntarily with any recommended protective services. The advisor might point out that such cooperation could enhance her ability to continue to live safely in her home and to retain control over her life. As an advisor, the attorney is obligated to advise Jane about the dangers and legal ramifications of driving when impaired. If the attorney thinks that Jane poses a real and immediate risk of causing serious harm to others through her use of her car, such that it would constitute a felony (such as vehicular assault or vehicular homicide), the attorney has a duty to report such a belief to law enforcement authorities. While such a report would not trigger around the clock guard or the confiscation of her car, it might bring yet another persuasive authority into her situation.

If the attorney has a reasonable belief that Jane lacks the capacity to make legal decisions on her own behalf, the attorney would be obligated to bring the matter to the attention of the county Probate Court. The court could on its own motion, or on the application of another party, conduct a hearing to determine if Jane needs the protection of the court in the form of a guardian. At this hearing, Jane also has the right to have an attorney represent her. As an advocate at such a proceeding, the attorney would urge the court to resolve all doubt regarding her competence in her favor, in order for her to retain as much decision-making authority over herself and her affairs as possible. If the court were to determine that Jane has some mental impairment that prevents her from providing for herself and her property, it would have to determine what type of guardianship protection is necessary. The court would only order full guardianship if no less restrictive alternative, such as a limited guardianship, is adequate to address the issue.

Wanda and Carl

If the physician who knows this family well were to respond to Wanda's phone call, he/she would likely question Wanda further about Carl's mental status, pain level, and ability to assist in his care. If possible, the physician would speak to Carl directly about his wishes regarding his care. If the physician believes that Wanda has not accurately reported Carl's wishes regarding care, an obligation to report suspected abuse, neglect, or exploitation would arise.

The duty of a physician to report suspected abuse, neglect, or exploitation is clear under Ohio's reporting statute.[90] This obligation mirrors the duty set forth for attorneys earlier in this article. Once the report is made, APS would be required to make a full investigation. After a full investigation, the APS worker will likely make a finding that abuse or neglect has occurred, and that one or both parties are in need of protective services.

Wanda and Carl require separate attorney representation, since their interests are significantly different. In this case, it will be difficult to sort out the victim from the perpetrator. Carl was physically and psychologically abusive to Wanda throughout their marriage. This probably engendered feelings of resentment and a strong desire to be free from his tyranny. Carl, who is now dependent and the probable victim of abuse and neglect at Wanda's hand, is still demanding and somewhat psychologically abusive.

It is clear that Carl cannot care for himself. Wanda is qualified to provide the care he needs under the circumstances. APS will probably recommend protective services, whether in the home or out of the home, which would involve an outlay of additional family resources. In this case, the attorneys representing Carl and Wanda respectively, would be required to vigorously protect the interests of the party represented. If a voluntary solution could be worked out, this could avoid any further legal action. Wanda cannot be required to provide physical care for Carl under any reading of the statutes. However, her financial resources are available to pay for this care since the law recognizes an obligation of one marriage partner to pay for the care of another if resources are available.

If a voluntary solution could not be worked out, and APS proposes an order for the involuntary provision of services to an incapacitated Carl, then all the due process rights outlined above are guaranteed to him. If Wanda also were named, then she too would have such protections. However, it is unclear what rights Wanda would have at a hearing for an involuntary order if she were not the subject of such an order, but merely the spouse whose resources would be used to accomplish the order. The attorney representing Wanda's interests would likely resist the execution of an order unless Wanda's liberty and property interests were considered.

While her current behavior cannot be ignored, it is likely that a prosecutor who might be reviewing this situation for prosecution would take Wanda's limitations and history of victimization into account. In the unlikely event that criminal charges were to be brought against Wanda, she would have all the Constitutional protections afforded to anyone charged with a crime, including: notice of all charges, the right to counsel, the right against self incrimination, the right to cross examine witnesses, the right to present evidence, and the right to have witnesses in her own behalf.

Brenda and Harriet

Brenda and Harriet are caught in a trap of economic, physical, social, emotional, and cognitive difficulties. The physical weariness and obvious depression that plague Brenda keeps her and her cognitively impaired mother in a state of social isolation. They are, because of these difficulties, either unable or unwilling to seek support from agencies that might provide some relief or assistance.

While not the focus of this case, the issue of abuse within the nursing homes that Brenda has worked at must be briefly addressed. The case scenario implies that Brenda has slapped or otherwise physically abused residents under her care in a work setting and that she has been "let go" or that she quit after accusations are made. It also implies that nothing is done to follow up on this situation. The law is clear that physical abuse in a nursing home or other residential care facility must be reported to, and investigated by, the Ohio Department of Health.[91] If the investigation reveals that an individual caring for residents in a long-term care facility has abused, neglected, or misappropriated a resident's funds, the Director of Health shall notify the individual, the facility employing the individual, the state Attorney General, County Prosecutor, and other appropriate law enforcement personnel.[92] Failure to report suspected abuse would result in civil fines and other sanctions against the facility. The vast majority of nursing home administrators consider abuse a very serious situation, will not tolerate it within the facility, and will not risk the penalties involved for failure to report.

In addition, the Director of Health is required to advise the Nurse Aide Registry of the finding against the individual. The notice must contain a "statement detailing the findings pertinent to the individual."[93] Facilities are required to query the Nurse Aide Registry when they hire an individual. Failure to do so could result in heightened liability for the facility and could result in survey deficiencies. Statutory provisions for addressing resident abuse, neglect, or exploitation vary among the states.

The investigatory process employed by the Department of Health is not flawless. The Department is often short staffed and investigations are slow. A query to retrieve statements in the records of the Nurse Aide Registry does not always result in a finding that the newly hired nurse aide had engaged in abusive activity at another facility. However, the system does work to keep the majority of abusive personnel from seeking and gaining employment. In addition, local authorities will usually pursue prosecutions of persons who engage in such behavior.

The case does not note that Brenda has physically abused her mother. However, she has threatened her mother with placement in a nursing facility or confinement to her room when she is not home to watch her. These threats probably produce anxiety in Harriet and thus are likely to meet the definition of "abuse" under the statute. This would bring Harriet within the strict definition of an abused person who is in need of protective services.

Harriet also appears to meet the definition of a person suffering from neglect under the statute, since she seems to have "the failure of an adult to provide for self the goods or services necessary to avoid physical harm, mental anguish, or mental illness or the failure to of a caretaker to provide such goods or services."[94] This again, could cause her to be classified as a person in need of protective services.

Harriet might also be classified as in need of protective services on the basis of exploitation because Brenda does not want to institutionalize her mother, although institutionalization would be in Harriet's best interests, it would deprive Brenda and her children of a place to live. Brenda also has allowed her children to steal money from Harriet's purse.

Harriet does not appear to have any real insight into her current situation. She wants to live in her own home even though it is to her own physical, financial, and emotional detriment. It is likely that she will resist any intervention and so a motion for an involuntary order for protective services will be filed and a hearing held. Harriet will have all the rights outlined above. Under the circumstances, Brenda also should seek an attorney of her own, since the findings of abuse, neglect, and exploitation could have significant impact on her as the perpetrator.

Harriet appears to be in need of a guardian to act in her best interests. If a proceeding were commenced to declare her incompetent and thus in need of guardian, a guardian *ad litem* might be appointed to make recommendations in this case. The guardian *ad litem* would fully investigate whether Harriet needed a guardian or whether some less restrictive alternative could be employed. The Probate Court where a hearing on the matter would be held will consider all that information. Harriet would have the right to an attorney and all the other legal protections outlined in the section on guardianships above.

This family is in great need for intervention before a tragedy results. While outside the scope of this discussion on elder abuse, a report to children's protective services within the jurisdiction should be made. It appears that these children are not receiving adequate supervision and care while their mother is away from home. Children of this age (i.e., 6 and 8) are too young to be left for long periods in the "care" of an incompetent grandmother. The fact that the children are stealing from Harriet is just one indication that they are not receiving adequate guidance and supervision. Brenda will need counsel to assist her in this situation as well, since a finding that the children are neglected could adversely affect her parental rights. The intervention of adult protective services and child protective services could do a great deal to assist this family in recovering an appropriate equilibrium.

CONCLUSION

An attorney involved in any of these cases must first ask the question, "Who is my client?" The duties and obligations of an attorney are defined by the answer to this one question. Attorneys are required to protect the confidences of and zealously represent the interests of the client even when a client appears to be engaging in risky behaviors. Some situations may present novel or complex issues with regard to the representation of the client, especially the client who may be incompetent, incapacitated, or mentally impaired in some way. In these cases the prudent attorneys should consult the Code and statutes that govern their conduct before proceeding.

The O.R.C. contains statutes that define elder abuse, neglect, and exploitation. These statutes were promulgated to protect vulnerable older adults. The statutes clearly define duties for a wide variety of professionals to report suspected situations involving abuse, neglect, or exploitation. They also set forth the responsibilities of the APS units within Ohio and the role of the court in such matters. Furthermore, the O.R.C. contains provisions to protect persons who are mentally impaired. Some provisions cover those persons who pose an immediate danger to themselves or others. Other provisions govern the appointment of guardians. All of these provisions carry due process safeguards, because they carry the consequence of the loss of some measure of liberty or freedom.

NOTES

1. The United States Census Bureau predicts a national increase in the older adult population. U.S. Census Bureau, Statistical Abstract of the United States, Table 1, Table 17 (119th ed. 1999).

2. In 1998, almost 31% of all seniors lived alone. U.S. Census (119th ed. 1999).

3. Lisa Nerenberg, *The Forgotten Victims of Elder Financial Crime and Abuse*, A Report and Recommendation 4 (The National Center on Elder Abuse, 1999) and Terrie Lewis, A Minnesota Comparative Family Law Symposium: *Fifty Ways to Exploit Your Grandmother: The Status of Financial Abuse of the Elderly in Minnesota*, 28 Wm. Mitchell L. Rev. 911 (2001).

4. Terrie Lewis, A Minnesota Comparative Family Law Symposium: *Fifty Ways to Exploit Your Grandmother: The Status of Financial Abuse of the Elderly in Minnesota*, 28 Wm. Mitchell L. Rev. 911 at p. 2 (2001).

5. Possible indicators of psychological/emotional abuse include: Helplessness, hesitation to talk openly, implausible stories, confusion or disorientation, anger, fear, withdrawal, depression, denial, and agitation. A.A.A.O.E and Elder Abuse Prevention, *http://www.oaktrees.org/elder/recog.shtml* (2001).

6. Possible Indicators of Financial Abuse include, but are not limited to,
- Unusual or inappropriate activity in bank statements;
- Signatures on checks, etc., that do not resemble the older person's signature, or signed when older person cannot write;
- Power of attorney given, or recent changes or creation of a Will, when the person is incapable of making such decisions;
- Unusual concern by caregiver that an excessive amount of money is being expended on the care of the older person;

- Numerous unpaid bills, overdue rent, when someone is supposed to be paying the bills for a dependent elder;
- Placement in nursing home or residential care facility which is not commensurate with alleged size of estate;
- Lack of amenities, such as TV, personal grooming items, appropriate clothing, that the estate can well afford;
- Missing personal belongings such as art, silverware, or jewelry; and
- Deliberate isolation, by a housekeeper, or an older adult from friends and family, resulting in the caregiver alone having total control.

A.A.A.O.E. and Elder Abuse Prevention, *http://www.oaktrees.org/elder/reocg.shtml* (2001).

7. Ohio Revised Code §2317.02 (A) covers privileged communications between an attorney and client. It states that an attorney shall not testify "concerning a communication made to the attorney by a client in that relation or the attorney's advice to a client, except that the attorney may testify by express consent of the client or, if the client is deceased, by the express consent of the surviving spouse or the executor of administrator of the estate of the deceased client and except that, if the client voluntarily testifies or . . . is deemed to have waived any testimonial privilege . . . " (1999).

8. "A lawyer should not accept compensation or any thing of value incident to his employment or services from one other than his client without the knowledge and consent of his client after full disclosure." Code of Professional Responsibility, EC 2-20 (1992).

9. Code of Professional Responsibility, Preface, Effective July 15, 1974.

10. Code of Professional Responsibility, Preface, Effective July 15, 1974.

11. Code of Professional Responsibility, Preface, Effective, July 15, 1974.

12. Model Rules, Preamble: A Lawyer's Responsibilities, 1989, American Bar Association (2002).

13. Model Rules, Preamble: A Lawyer's Responsibilities, 1989, American Bar Association. (2002).

14. Code of Professional Responsibility, Canon 4 (1992).

15. Code of Professional Responsibility, DR 4-101 (1992).

16. Code of Professional Responsibility, EC 4-2 (1992).

17. Chapter 29 of the Ohio Revised Code codifies criminal offenses. The elements of a crime are carefully defined. When interpreting these statutes one must carefully cite the specific language of the statute and narrowly construe it.

18. *People v. Fentress*, 425 N.Y.S. 2d 485, 491 (1980).

19. ABA Commission on ethics and Professional Responsibility, Informal Opinion 83-1500 (1983).

20. Code of Professional Responsibility, EC 7-1 (1992).

21. Code of Professional Responsibility, EC 7-1 (1992).

22. Code of Professional Responsibility, EC 7-2 (1992).

23. Code of Professional Responsibility, EC 7-3 (1992).

24. Code of Professional Responsibility, EC 7-11 (1992).

25. Code of Professional Responsibility, EC 7-12 (1992).

26. Code of Professional Responsibility, EC 7-12 (1992).

27. Code of Professional Responsibility, EC 7-12 (1992).

28. Model Rules 1.14 (a), American Bar Association (2002).

29. Comment on Model Rule 1.14, American Bar Association (2002).

30. Model Rules 1.14 (b), American Bar Association (2002).

31. Bart J. Collopy, Autonomy in Long-term Care: Some Crucial Distractions, *The Gerontologist, 28,* 10-17 (1988).

32. Marshall B. Kapp and Arthur Bigot, Geriatrics and the Law: *Informed Consent and Telling-Truth* (1985)

33. Ohio Revised Code §2111.01 (D) (1999).

34. Ohio Revised Code §5101.60 (B) (1999).

35. Ohio Revised Code §5101.60 (A) (1999).

36. Ohio Revised Code §5101.60 (M) (1999).

37. Ohio Revised Code §5101.60 (K) (1999).

38. Ohio Revised Code §5101.60 (G) (1999).

39. *State v. Flontek,* 82 OS3d 10, 693 NE2d 767.

40. Ohio Revised Code §2919.21 (B) (2) (1999).

41. Ohio Revised Code §2919.21 (D) (1999).

42. For example see Ky. Rev. Stat. Ann. §209.060 (2002) and Nevada Rev. Stat. Ann §200.5093 (2002) .

43. Article IV, §2 (B) (1) (g), the "Modern Courts Amendment of 1968" states that the Ohio "Supreme Court shall have original jurisdiction in the following: . . . [A]dmission to the practice of law, the discipline of persons so admitted, and all other matters relating to the practice of law."

44. Ohio Revised Code§5101.61 (D) provides that "Any person with reasonable cause to believe that an adult is suffering abuse, neglect, or exploitation who makes a report pursuant to this section or testifies in any administrative or judicial proceeding arising from such report . . . shall be immune from civil or criminal liability on account of such investigation, report, testimony . . . unless the person has acted in bad faith or with malicious purpose." (2002).

45. Ohio Revised Code §5101.61 (A)(6)(g)(ii) (1999).

46. Ohio Revised Code §5101.61 (C)(1)-(4) (1999).

47. Ohio Revised Code §5101.99 (1999).

48. Ohio Revised Code §5101.62 (1999).

49. Ohio Revised Code §5101.62 (1999).

50. Ohio Revised Code §5101.63 (1999).

51. Ohio Revised Code §5101.63 (1999).

52. Ohio Revised Code §5101.62 (1999).

53. Ohio Revised Code §5101.64 (1999).

54. Ohio Revised Code §5101.65 (1999).

55. Ohio Revised Code §5101.60 (I) (1999).

56. Ohio Revised Code §5101.67 (1999).

57. Ohio Revised Code §5101.67 (1999).

58. Ohio Revised Code §5101.67 (B) (1999).

59. Ohio Revised Code §5101.67 (E) (1999).

60. Ohio Revised Code §5101.67 (C) (1999).

61. Model Rule 1.14 (b), American Bar Association (2002).

62. Guardianship Law Safeguards Personal Rights Yet Protects Vulnerable Elderly, Akron Law Review, Vol. 24, p.166 (1990).

63. Guardianship Law Safeguards Personal Rights Yet Protects Vulnerable Elderly, Akron Law Review, Vol. 24, p.162 (1990).

64. Ohio Revised Code §2111.01 (A) (1999).

65. Ohio Revised Code §2111.02 (A) and (B) (1) (1999).

66. Ohio Revised Code §2111.01 (D) (1999).

67. 1990 Guardianship Law Safeguards Personal Rights Yet Protects Vulnerable Elderly, Akron Law Review, Vol. 24, p. 169 (1990).

68. 1990 Guardianship Law Safeguards Personal Rights Yet Protects Vulnerable Elderly, Akron Law Review, Vol. 24, p. 169 (1990).

69. Ohio Revised Code §2111.041(A) (1)-(4) (1999).

70. Ohio Revised Code §2111.041(B) (1999).

71. Ohio Revised Code §2111.02 (C) (7) (1999).

72. Ohio Revised Code §2111.50 (A)-(E) (1999).

73. Ohio Revised Code §2111.50 (A) (1) (1999)

74. Ohio Revised Code §5122.01 (B)(1) and (B)(3) (1999).

75. Ohio Revised Code §5122.01 (B)(2) (1999)

76. Ohio Revised Code §5122.05 (C) (1) & (2) (1999).

77. Nina Santo, *"Breaking the Silence: Strategies for Combating Elder Abuse in California,"* 31 McGeorge L. Rev. 801, at p. 3, (Spring 2000) and Elder Abuse: A Decade of Shame and Inaction, Hearing Before the Subcommittee on Health and Long-Term Care of the House Select Committee on Aging, 101st Congress, 2nd Session 3, at p. 97 (1990).

78. Nina Santo, *"Breaking the Silence: Strategies for Combating Elder Abuse in California,"* 31 McGeorge L. Rev. 801, at p. 3, (Spring 2000).

79. Ohio Revised Code §2929.21 (D) (1999)

80. Ohio Revised Code §5101.60 (A) (1999).

81. Ohio Revised Code §2903.11 states that "No person shall knowingly . . . cause serious physical harm to another . . . whoever violates this section is guilty of felonious assault, a felony of the second degree." The comments on this section indicates that the "section does not distinguish among persons and, except with respect to deadly weapons and dangerous ordnance, is not based on the means used to commit the offense . . . the relative gravity of this offense and the three lesser assault offenses following it is graded according to three factors: the degree of culpability; the seriousness of the actual or potential harm involved; and whether or not a deadly weapon is used. . . . This section is a lesser-included offense to attempted murder, which is a felony of the first degree (1999).

82. The Domestic Violence statute, Ohio Revised Code §2919.25 states that "[N]o person shall knowingly cause or attempt to cause physical harm to a family or household member. . . . No person shall recklessly cause serious physical harm to a family or household member. . . . No person, by threat of force, shall knowingly cause a family or household member to believe that the offender will cause imminent physical harm to the family or household member." The offense is graded based on whether harm was actually caused and whether this is a first or subsequent offense (1999).

83. Aggravated Menacing, Ohio Revised Code §2903.21 is defined as "knowingly caus[ing] another to believe that the offender will cause serious physical harm to the person or property of such other person. Aggravated Menacing is a misdemeanor of the first degree" (1999).

84. Ohio Revised Code §2929.21 (B) (1) and (C) (1) (1999).

85. Ohio Revised Code §2929.21 (B) (2) and (C) (2) (1999).

86. Misuse of Credit Cards, ORC §2913.21 (B) "No person, with purpose to defraud, shall do any of the following: (1) Obtain control over a credit card as a security for a debt; (2) Obtain property or services by the use of a credit card, in one or more transactions, knowing or having reasonable cause to believe that the card has expired or been revoked, or was obtained, is retained, or is being used in violation of law; . . .

(D)(4) If the victim of the offense is an elderly person or disabled adult, and if the offense involves a violation of division (B)(1) or (2) of this section, division (D)(4) of this section, a violation of division (B)(1) or (2) of this section is a felony of the fifth degree" (1999).

87. *State v. Guilford*, Ohio App., Lexis 214 (1998).

88. Forgery . . . ORC§2913.31:(A), states in part "No person, with purpose to defraud, or knowing that the person is facilitating a fraud, shall do any of the following: (1) Forge any writing of another without the other person's authority; (2) Forge any writing so that it purports to be genuine when it actually is spurious, or to be the act of another who did not authorize that act, or to have been executed at a time or place or with terms different from what in fact was the case, or to be a copy of an original when no such original existed; (3) Utter, or possess with purpose to utter, any writing that the person knows to have been forged. . . . Whoever violates division (A) of this section is guilty of forgery" (1999).

89. For example, Ohio Revised Code §2919.26 sets forth the requirements for the issuance of temporary protective orders. These orders are designed to protect the victim and other family and household members from retaliation by the alleged perpetrator (1999).

90. Ohio Revised Code §5101.61 (A)(6)(g)(ii) outlines the professionals who are required to make reports of suspected abuse, neglect or exploitation to the County Department of Jobs and Family Services (1999).

91. Ohio Revised Code §3721.22 (A) states "No licensed health professional who knows or suspects that a resident has been abused or neglected, or that a resident's property has been misappropriated, by any individual used by a long-term care facility or residential care facility to provide services to residents shall fail to report that knowledge or suspicion to the director of health." Abuse as used in this section is defined as "knowingly causing physical harm or recklessly causing serious physical harm to a resident by physical contact with a resident or by the use of physical or chemical restraint, medication, or isolation as punishment, for staff convenience . . . or in amounts that preclude habilitation and treatment." Ohio Revised Code §3721.21 (C) (1999).

92. Ohio Revised Code §3721.23 (C) (1) (1999).

93. Ohio Revised Code §3721.23 (C) (1) (a) (1999).

94. Ohio Revised Code §5101.60 (K) (1999).

Elder Abuse:
The Physician's Perspective

John F. McGreevey, Jr., MD

SUMMARY. The various forms of elder abuse and neglect affect large numbers of older adults in the United States. Physicians have an ethical and, in most states, legal role in recognition and intervention where elder mistreatment is suspected. A number of risk factors have been identified, usually focusing on patient vulnerability, as well as caregiver and financial factors. Additional complicating elements include caregiver stress and burden, the patient's cognitive abilities and decisional capacity, and pre-existing psychosocial concerns aggravated by health and financial issues. The three cases discussed in this paper represent a range of these concerns. They present serious challenges to physicians and other health care providers. Awareness of legal and ethical concerns, attention to communication, and principles of geriatric care can enhance the physician's ability to address these situations. *[Article copies available for a fee from The Haworth Document Delivery Service: 1-800-HAWORTH. E-mail address: <docdelivery@haworthpress.com> Website: <http://www.HaworthPress.com> © 2005 by The Haworth Press, Inc. All rights reserved.]*

KEYWORDS. Elder abuse, role of physicians, diagnosis, clinical management

INTRODUCTION AND OVERVIEW

The spectrum of elder abuse includes physical abuse, physical neglect, psychological abuse, psychological neglect, sexual abuse, finan-

John F. McGreevey, Jr. is affiliated with the Office of Geriatric Medicine, Medical College of Ohio, Toledo, Ohio.

[Haworth co-indexing entry note]: "Elder Abuse: The Physician's Perspective." McGreevey, Jr., John F. Co-published simultaneously in *Clinical Gerontologist* (The Haworth Press, Inc.) Vol. 28, No. 1/2, 2005, pp. 83-103; and: *The Clinical Management of Elder Abuse* (ed: Georgia J. Anetzberger) The Haworth Press, Inc., 2005, pp. 83-103. Single or multiple copies of this article are available for a fee from The Haworth Document Delivery Service [1-800-HAWORTH, 9:00 a.m. - 5:00 p.m. (EST). E-mail address: docdelivery@haworthpress.com].

cial victimization, and self-neglect. Some authors have suggested that the term elder maltreatment might more accurately reflect the broad range of occurrences in which an older adult is victimized. Various studies have estimated that between 500,000 to as many as two million older adults in this country have experienced abuse in a year (Department of Health and Human Services, 1998; Lachs & Pillemer, 1995). Elder abuse and self-neglect both have been associated with increased mortality, even when adjusted for co-existing illness (Lachs, Williams, O'Brien, Pillemer, & Charlson, 1998). Underrecognition and under-reporting of elder abuse remain significant concerns with estimates that as few as 20 percent of cases are ever actually reported (Silverman & Hudson, 2000). Physicians may see many of the sequela of elder abuse and are, in most states, legally responsible for reporting abuse and neglect. Despite this fact, physicians report a fairly small percentage of identified cases of elder abuse (Rosenblatt, Cho, & Dorrance, 1996). There are several potential reasons for this fact, including difficulties with definition and recognition, as well as difficulties with intervention and follow-up.

Overt physical abuse is generally easier to define than various forms of neglect where issues of caregiver responsibility, underlying patient condition, and the patient's wishes and capacity for self-determination may open matters to more interpretation. However, recognition may still present challenges. In the case of physical abuse, the physician must obviously have the opportunity to see the patient and must recognize that injuries do not fit the described event or that multiple injurious events are happening. The injuries should be placed in the context of the frailty and illness of the patient. For example, a patient who is very frail can develop bruises without significant trauma. A patient with severe osteoporosis can develop a bone fracture during routine care and activity. The pattern and frequency of injury become important. The identification of bruises or injuries of various ages or injuries that don't fit the described events are good examples. All injuries should be objectively described and documented, using photographs where appropriate (Lachs & Pillemer, 1995; Silverman & Hudson, 2000; Harrell et al., 2002; Kennedy, 2000). Next, the physician should interview the patient alone for information about the events, interview the caregiver separately, and observe the nature of the interactions between the patient and caregiver. If there is suspicion of physical abuse, the physician has three responsibilities. First, observations should be accurately and specifically documented. Second, an assessment should be made of whether the patient is in immediate danger and whether he or she should be hospitalized.

Finally, suspicions of abuse should be reported to Adult Protective Services. In Ohio, as in most states, this is required by law. A proof that abuse has occurred is not necessary to make a report and health professionals are provided with civil immunity when they report abuse (Lachs & Pillemer, 1995; Ohio Revised Code. Section 5101.60-5101.62, 2000).

Psychological abuse, neglect, and self-neglect can be more difficult to identify. Some studies have found that neglect and self-neglect are the most commonly reported forms of elder maltreatment (Department of Health and Human Services, 1998; Silverman & Hudson, 2000). Despite that, physicians often have difficulties determining the boundary between difficult circumstances and neglect. Suspicions of psychological abuse and neglect are viewed in the context of the relationship. For example, if two people have always had an argumentative relationship, the physician may find it difficult to determine that this has developed into psychological abuse. In this situation, the increasing vulnerability and care needs of either person may be the defining factor. It is also difficult to define the point when an individual crosses the line from making unsafe choices to self-neglect. Is it ageist to say that a forty-year-old may choose poor self-care and health habits but an eighty-year-old may not do the same? The key factors in making this determination would likely be patient vulnerability and decisional capacity, as well as the degree to which the situation is truly one the patient has chosen.

Additional barriers to identification of maltreatment include a patient's inability to relate events and the health care professional's dependence on caregivers for information about events occurring at home. Patients who can relate events may be reluctant to do so because they may not want to be removed from the home situation despite the difficulties (Kennedy, 2000). They may fear reprisal from the abuser. In addition, physicians and other health care professionals may be reluctant to raise the issue of abuse or neglect. Quality geriatric care generally involves establishment of a trusting relationship with patients and their caregivers. Reporting may create more of an adversarial relationship between physician and patient or physician and caregiver. This is more likely to be a concern in cases of self-neglect or in situations of poor care from an exhausted, overwhelmed caregiver, as opposed to occurrences of overt and deliberate victimization.

The presence of chronic disease is another complicating circumstance. Generally, chronic debility due to illness is considered a risk factor for elder abuse, although there is not total agreement about that fact (Lachs & Pillemer, 1995). However, patient vulnerability due to disease is usually one of the key features in the definition of elder abuse and neglect, so it would be likely for vulnerable older adults to be heavily represented in any study of elder abuse. In the presence of a degenerative disease it can be difficult to determine whether a person's deterioration is due to the inexorable course of the disease or due to poor care. With the demented person, poor recall of events, as well as the presence of delusions or inaccurate perceptions, can make the task of the interviewer even more difficult. For example, how does one know if the person with delusions of theft is actually getting robbed? Nutritional problems are common as a dementia progresses, making it difficult to know when a person is losing weight due to disease as opposed to poor provision of nutrition. The goals for intervention in such a situation may change as the disease progresses. In these instances, specific caregiver descriptions of feeding efforts and other care problems may help the physician or other interviewer gain insight into the patient's environment.

It takes time to sort through all of the issues raised above. Unfortunately, in most physicians' office settings time is at a premium. The very patients that are at highest risk for abuse are those who also require extra time for management of their medical concerns. Physicians also may feel nihilistic about the outcome of making a referral. As a result, the right questions may never be asked. Regardless of these difficulties in recognition and intervention of elder maltreatment, physicians have an ethical obligation to take on this task. In addition, they have a legal obligation to report elder abuse in most states (Lachs & Pillemer, 1995).

The existing medical literature on elder abuse focuses largely on identification of risk and recognition of abuse. There are fewer guidelines for intervention and follow-up after a report has been filed.

Recognition begins with (1) an understanding of patient and caregiver risk factors, and (2) knowledge of common warnings of an abusive situation. Abused persons have been described as most likely women, over age 80, and experiencing some physical or cognitive frailty due to one or more diseases. However, some studies that have adjusted for larger numbers of older women have not found women at higher risk to be victims of elder abuse and have shown a more heterogeneous picture of victims of abuse. The classical symptoms above seem to be more accurate when describing victims of neglect. Cognitive impairment and depression also emerge as risk factors. In some profiles of abusers, women are more heavily represented in cases of neglect and men are more heavily represented in other forms of abuse. The former may reflect the greater numbers of women involved in caregiver roles. Abusers tend to be younger than the abused, with the greatest age difference occurring in cases of financial exploitation. They are usually related to the victim of abuse. Other risk factors for abuse include a history of substance abuse on the part of the abuser, financial dependency of the abuser upon the victim, history of mental illness in the abuser, and history of violence on the part of the abuser (Lachs & Pillemer, 1995; Silverman & Hudson, 2000; Kennedy, 2000).

Signs of physical abuse have been reviewed above. However, the physician should not wait for obvious evidence before considering abuse. The American Medical Association released guidelines in 1992 recommending that physicians routinely ask patients questions about whether they had ever been hurt, coerced, molested, threatened or neglected. Questions about financial victimization also should be asked (American Medical Association, 1992). In addition, signs of caregiver exhaustion and frustration can be identified and hopefully addressed before abuse or neglect occurs. As noted earlier, observations of patient-caregiver interactions can be illuminating. During the course of a visit one may witness evidence of frustration and impatience on the part of a caregiver. The caregiver may dominate the interaction excessively, not allowing the patient to express him or herself. Statements that overly belittle the patient and fearful reactions on the part of the patient also should raise concerns. Frequently missed appointments and requests for psychotropic drugs that seem excessive for the patient's described symptoms provide additional clues (Kennedy, 2000).

To continue the assessment one needs to speak with the patient alone to get his or her perceptions on what is occurring and to understand their insight into the situation. The caregiver should be interviewed separately as well. Ideally, this will have occurred on an ongoing basis. Depending on the clinical setting and the availability of a geriatric care team, interviews may be done by a variety of professionals. During this interview one can explore the caregiver's perception of how things are going. It is important to be as specific as possible about the patient-caregiver relationship, including identification of specific sources of distress and the response to them. For example, if the patient is losing weight, the interviewer should obtain details about feeding efforts and strategies. This will help distinguish between situations where a best effort is being made unsuccessfully and those in which neglect may be present. These discussions will provide another opportunity to assess the degree of caregiver fatigue and frustration. It will also be helpful to watch for signs of general regard and empathy for the patient on the part of the caregiver. The interviewer can begin to identify the caregiver who is frustrated, angry, or exhausted, being alert for comments that would signal the possibility of abuse or neglect and learning more about the relationship between caregiver and patient.

The information elicited during the caregiver interview is not intended to trick or trap the caregiver, but to identify problems in the relationship that may lead to abuse and neglect or to identify abuse or neglect that has occurred. The ideal goal of the physician is to help both patient and caregiver, though the prime duty of the physician is to the patient. The physician and team members can hopefully improve the situation by helping the caregiver to develop some insight and perspective on what is occurring. Problems should be discussed not in a confrontational style, but with empathy for the caregiver's predicament. Opportunities for caregiver counseling and education, as well as changes in the care plan can be presented and explored. In those circumstances where there is criminal intent, such as in financial victimization, confrontation may be necessary and law enforcement agencies are more likely to be involved at an earlier stage (Lachs & Pillemer, 1995; Silverman & Hudson, 2000; Kennedy, 2000).

Each physician should know his or her state laws for the reporting of elder abuse. As noted above, if there is suspicion of abuse, reporting may be mandated. Ideally, the referral can be framed as a method for engaging all available problem-solving resources as opposed to an accusation of wrongdoing. Adult Protective Services should be identified as a support agency, although the legal mandate of reporting abuse and neglect also should be reinforced. Reporting does not end the physician's responsibility, as there will be ongoing needs for reassessment, follow-up, and counseling.

The cases under discussion in this paper focus more on neglect than intentional physical abuse. The issues identified include self-neglect, physical neglect, psychological abuse and potential financial victimization. None of these cases involve overt criminal intent. Instead they illustrate the complex biopsychosocial matrix in which abuse and neglect can occur. The discussion will focus upon the circumstances in which a physician might become involved with each patient and caregiver, the manner in which abuse might be identified, and possible interventions and follow-up. In each case, the prime duty to protect and care for the patient is foremost, but the opportunities to assist both patient and caregiver also are recognized. The role of the physician in assessment and management of elder mistreatment will have many facets. First, the physician may be a primary contact for patients and caregivers and so may be in the best position to recognize signs of abuse and neglect. He or she may best assess when the patient's clinical condition can be explained on the basis of identifiable conditions and when poor care or overt mistreatment are possibilities. He or she will then be the person in the best position to make a referral to Adult Protective Services. The physician also will have the responsibility of minimizing vulnerability by optimally managing injuries and medical conditions. Evaluation and management may include assessment of cognitive capabilities when decisional capacity plays a role in the patient's situation. Finally, the physician will have an ongoing responsibility in the management of the patient during and after any ongoing investigations of abuse and neglect.

JANE

Self-neglect is one of the more difficult dimensions of elder abuse to address. Common presenting problems include poor self-care and nutrition, living in an unsafe environment, and allowing for animal infestation, all of which are at least considered in Jane's case. The elements of evaluation of self-neglect include the determination of whether the situation is volitional, whether the patient has the capacity for self-determination, and whether the safety issues rise to the level of reportablility. A key determinant to the latter question is whether the patient meets the criteria for being a vulnerable adult. In the state of Ohio this definition would be "any person sixty years of age or older within this state who is handicapped by the infirmities of aging or who has a physical or mental impairment which prevents the person from providing for the person's own care or protection, and who resides in an independent living arrangement" (Ohio Revised Code. Section 5101.60-5101.62, 2000). In the absence of physical or mental impairment, it is not clear what the "infirmities of aging" might be. As part of this assessment, the physician has the responsibility for evaluation and management of medical conditions that may be increasing the patient's vulnerability. Self-neglect strongly tests the balance between autonomy and beneficence and therefore presents conflicting ethical duties for the health care professional.

Jane's story poses a number of dilemmas. Because Jane is not one to seek assistance, it is unlikely that she would see a physician until there was a crisis or catastrophe, most likely a hospitalization from acute illness or injury. Unfortunately, there is no one who would be likely to check on her in her current situation, snowed in with a limited food supply. There is, in fact, a strong possibility that Jane would, at some point, be found deceased in her home. If a physician encounter did occur, it would most likely find Jane acutely ill or injured and in the hospital setting. Acute concerns might need to be addressed first. If she were healthy enough for interaction, she would most likely be somewhat wary and guarded. Jane's story suggests a mistrust of institutions and officials. It is unlikely that she would accept a recommendation to move to a more protected environment if such a suggestion were made. As she is evaluated and treated, the health care team may begin to face some of the concerns regarding her home environment.

Key tasks confronting Jane's physician will include the establishment of a working relationship, assessment of possible medical issues, and the question of whether there is sufficient evidence of self-neglect to warrant a referral to Adult Protective Services. The latter question will involve a determination of whether Jane is a vulnerable adult. This will require some awareness of her decisional capacity. To that end it will be important to establish whether Jane has insight into her current situation and condition, whether she understands the choices she's making and the consequences of these decisions, and whether she can demonstrate values underlying the decision and communicate this in some fashion. Whether or not she makes the decision the health care team wants is not relevant in assessing her ability to decide (Kennedy, 2000).

Jane's current lifestyle is one of social isolation. Indications are that she prefers things that way. Throughout her life she has managed without the assistance of others and has apparently resented other people, even those who are well-meaning. Some of these feelings about others may have originated in her younger years when she had to be more guarded and when openness might have been dangerous. That aside, there is an established pattern of avoidance of others, a general disdain for other people and a specific lack of interest in advice or help from outsiders. She exhibits some signs of an antisocial personality.

Establishing a physician-patient relationship will be somewhat difficult. As noted, she has little trust in the health care system. Treating acute problems may go relatively well, but assessment and follow-up of chronic concerns is likely to be frustrating. At this juncture, Jane is unlikely to believe that she needs help. This attitude and the decisions she has been making about her living situation seem consistent with the choices she has made throughout her life. Developing a physician-patient relationship involves learning what her values, decisions, and priorities are and respecting them. It is then important to see if mutual goals can be established. The physician can clarify his or her role and offer advice and recommendations, recognizing that these may clash with Jane's priorities. A good starting point is to focus on the mutual goal of optimizing her independence. If rapport can be established, Jane might be willing to discuss some of the issues of concern to her health care providers. Any approach is likely to be an uphill battle, but an attitude that respects Jane's intelligence is more likely to be successful than one that is condescending or authoritative.

As acute problems are stabilized, an assessment should be done for medical problems that may be contributing to Jane's poor function. In the absence of a working furnace, she might be using additional methods to stay warm, including unsafe practices, like overuse of space heaters and the use of an oven or stove to heat a room, raising concerns about carbon monoxide toxicity as well as the danger of fire. Also, the inadequate heating puts Jane at risk for hypothermia, which could present with cognitive, perceptual, and gait problems. Alcohol use is an additional risk factor for hypothermia.

It is important to screen for systemic illnesses, such as hypothyroidism, that might add to her functional problems. Her vision and its potential for correction need to be assessed. Several additional questions are raised by the case presentation. There is the question of alcoholism. The patient's apathy and lack of interest in things around her suggest the possibility of depression. The memory difficulties described earlier could be a sign of dementia or may relate to alcohol use, depression, or other undiagnosed medical problems.

Jane's assessment should begin with her life history, in order to establish rapport and to learn about her background and living situation. This interview also can help the physician gain awareness of her memory and insight. As the focus of the interview shifts to Jane's current living situation, questions can be directed to how she is managing at home. Her ability to manage her personal finances, for example, would support her ability to cognitively manage independent living (Barbas & Wilde, 2001). The medical history and physical evaluation should include focus on constitutional and nonspecific symptoms, which are more common signs of chronic illness in older adults.

Assessment of her alcohol use should begin with questions about her quantitative alcohol use (drinks per day, days of drinking per week, episodes of binge drinking), her insight into the role that alcohol plays in her life, and a discussion of the medical consequences of alcohol use. Tools such as the Michigan Alcohol Screening Test-Geriatric scale, the CAGE questionnaire, or possibly both, could provide further insight into the impact of alcohol on her life (More, Seeman, Morgenstern, Beck, & Reuben, 2002).

Depression screening also should be included. Simple questions about depressed mood and anhedonia would provide an opening. The Geriatric Depression Scale also would be a useful tool, although Jane's outlook on life might inflate her score (Yesavage, 2001).

Identification of Jane's cognitive capacity is a critical task. Many physicians are not trained in evaluating decisional capacity. Training physicians to understand the standards for evaluating capacity can improve interrater agreement (Marson, Earnst, Jamil, Bartolucci, & Harrell, 2000). These standards, mentioned earlier, include the ability to understand a situation, apply a set of values to a choice, demonstrate a choice, understand the consequences of a choice, and communicate that choice (Kennedy, 2000; Barbas & Wilde, 2001).

Performance on cognitive testing provides supportive information, but the most important information comes from the functional ability demonstrated by the patient. For most clinicians the Folstein Mini-Mental State would be the initial test of Jane's cognitive ability (Folstein, Folstein, & McHugh, 1975). However, this test is probably of limited value in determining Jane's decisional capacity.

Physicians do not have simple, readily available tools to establish a person's capacity to live independently. The patient's insight and awareness of his or her situation is an indicator of ability to exercise judgment (Barbas & Wilde, 2001). Impairment of spatial orientation and judgment, as well as lack of awareness of deficits increases concerns about patient safety. There is evidence that executive function, the ability to think abstractly, plan, initiate a sequence of actions, and monitor results, is a key determinant of decisional capacity and ability to function independently (Kennedy, 2000; Kennedy, 2002; Royall, Mahurin, & Gray, 1992; Schindler, Ramchandi, Mathews, & Podell, 1995; Royall, Cabello, & Polk, 1998).

Executive dysfunction is usually associated with frontal lobe dysfunction but has been described in subcortical dementias. In one recent study, tests associated with executive function, as well as some measures of verbal skills and comprehension, showed high correlation with decisional capacity (Earnst, Marson, & Harrell, 2002). People with executive dysfunction are more likely to have problems with activities of daily living (ADL) and instrumental activities of daily living (IADL) and, therefore, are more likely to have problems maintaining independence. Executive function has been correlated with level of independence in one's living situation. The clock drawing test, ability to follow sequential instructions (Luria 3-fist test), word list generation, and alternating sequence tasks, such as Trail Making B, can be helpful in evaluating executive function at the bedside or in the office. A specific tool, the Executive Interview also has been developed (Kennedy, 2000; Royall et al., 1992; Schindler et al., 1995; Royall et al., 1998). Psychiatric and neuropsychological referrals will be indicated if the physician is not well-versed in this sort of determination or if there is persistent doubt about capacity.

Again, although accurate diagnosis is important, the patient's functional status will be more important than the specific diagnosis in establishing her decisional capacity. Consultation with occupational therapy will assist in establishing her ability to carry out ADLs and IADLs and may lead to additional therapeutic recommendations. Social service should be involved early in the hospitalization to assist in counseling Jane, and to help in making plans.

If Jane is insightful and aware of her current situation and is making reasoned choices that are consistent with the choices she has made throughout her life, her decision, while possibly unwise, should be respected. The physician should reinforce his or her willingness to work with Jane to meet her goals and should, at the same time, reinforce the goal of each intervention as helping Jane to maintain her optimal independence. It is also important to recognize the limits of what we can provide and to acknowledge and respect her intelligence. Presenting oneself as an all-knowing expert would be especially unsuccessful here.

If Jane does not have the capacity to understand her current situation and this is due to an irreversible problem, such as a dementia, the question of where she lives becomes a legal issue referred to the probate court, since she has no one that would be a surrogate decision-maker. The physician's responsibility is then the documentation and reporting of the evidence of Jane's capacity as well as Jane's ongoing care needs.

The physician also must face the decision of whether to make a report to Adult Protective Services. As noted, if there is a suspicion of neglect, the physician is required to make a report. Two key features in Jane's case would be the presence of risk to the patient and the evidence of patient vulnerability. The information provided certainly suggests a person at risk, given the inadequate heating, danger of fire, poor access to nutrition, and hygiene issues. Five feet of snow represents an extraordinary circumstance that would pose danger for many people and is probably irrelevant to this determination. There is also significant evidence of patient vulnerability in Jane's forgetfulness and visual impairment. While her current living situation may be one of her choosing, it is the change in her health that has threatened her ability to live in the situation safely. There are indicators that her health problems may prevent her from providing for her own care and protection as defined by law in Ohio (Lachs, Williams et al., 1998). From that standpoint, there is probably sufficient suspicion of self-neglect to mandate the involvement of Adult Protective Services, if a referral has not already been made. This should be done openly, with acknowledgement of the legal obligation and reinforcement of the advocacy role played by Adult Protective Services. This referral may be met with mistrust on Jane's part, but open discussion may help maintain the working relationship.

It is likely that Jane is going to want to return to her home setting and, unfortunately, it is unlikely that she will accept a great deal of help. Post-discharge follow-up should include the Adult Protective Services referral, consideration of in-home services, and medical follow up. Office visits should be encouraged if transportation can be arranged. If Jane is unwilling or unable to come to the office, home visits should be considered, depending on Jane's willingness to accept these. There is every possibility that Jane will return to a high-risk living situation and we may need to respect her decision to do so. Ongoing attempts should be made to negotiate a continuing working relationship with her.

WANDA AND CARL

The relationship presented in the story of Wanda and Carl is complex, in that Wanda has been a victim of abuse throughout much of her life and now stands poised to become the abuser in the relationship. The physician's role in this case can include that of being Carl's physician, Wanda's physician, or the physician to both of them.

Carl's physician would need to focus on his well-being and his wishes for care, regardless of the fact that he is not a sympathetic character. As presented here, he is now terminally ill and so his goals for care are likely to focus on comfort and quality of life opposed to prolongation of life. Part of the physician's assessment involves establishing Carl's current health status and the degree to which he is to care for himself. In addition, it is important to evaluate his current symptoms and therapy and whether effective palliation is being accomplished.

The available information suggests that Carl can do very little without assistance. This puts certain responsibilities on Wanda if she chooses to accept the role as his primary caregiver. In Ohio a caretaker is described as "the person assuming the responsibility for the care of an adult on a voluntary basis, by contract, through receipt of payment for care, as a result of a family relationship, or by order of a court of competent jurisdiction" (Ohio Revised Code Section 5101.60-5101.62, 2000). Care plans must focus on what Carl wants and does not want, but at the same time Wanda can make decisions about what she can or cannot do and whether she can accept the role of being Carl's caregiver. Although Carl has the right to make the decisions in his care, he does not have the right to make unilateral decisions that infringe upon Wanda's rights and health, such as refusing help and insisting that she be his sole caregiver (Kennedy, 2000). Abandonment is not an option, but there may be alternatives to the current situation.

It is unclear how much of the background of Wanda and Carl's relationship the physician would know at this time. Carl's social history would hopefully include some discussions of his personality and approach to life. Prior discussions with Wanda may have provided the physician with some insight into their relationship.

A person who feels trapped in the caregiver relationship and who cannot feel any affection or compassion for the care receiver presents significant potential for abuse and neglect. This person will have trouble meeting the needs of the patient. Discussions with Wanda, as Carl's wife and caregiver, should include information about their marital relationship and descriptions of her day-to-day experiences as a caregiver. Information about the past abuse might be shared openly by Wanda, revealed by other family members, or not revealed at all.

The physician should be open to signs of increased frustration and exhaustion that may lead Wanda to approach the threshold of neglect or abuse. Questions about day-to-day difficulties and the physical and emotional demands of caring for Carl provide logical openings to explore Wanda's feelings. The discussion can then focus on specific questions about how far her frustration has taken her. From there, specific occurrences can be discussed and it is here that specific evidence of imminent or occurring abuse or neglect might emerge (Lachs & Pillemer, 1995; Silverman & Hudson, 2000; Kennedy, 2000). Ideally, these discussions would have taken place on an ongoing basis and hopefully would have revealed problems before an actual reportable or dangerous event.

Conversations with Wanda also should include a review of Carl's health status and function. Wanda's reactions to Carl are influenced by a lifetime of abuse, but the context of Carl's behavior may have changed. Wanda may benefit from the insight that the current demands upon her are not necessarily a manifestation of the abusive and domineering personality she knows but may be related to the impact of the illness on Carl. This is an important distinction. It is analogous to the caregiver of a demented person who has difficulty distinguishing between whether the patient is purposefully being difficult or is unable to cooperate.

It might be useful to explore Wanda's reasons for staying in the relationship over the years and remaining the primary caregiver now. The case narrative suggests she stayed in the relationship because of a combination of religious obligation and the feeling that she has no other options. She may feel that she is trapped in this situation and she may have not experienced a sense of having choices or options. Her self-esteem appears to be very low. In addition, she may have faced some genuine financial obstacles to leaving Carl. These reasons may still be key factors in her decisions. She also may look at the current situation as a chance to prove her value to Carl or to finally have the upper hand in the relationship. She may not be consciously aware of these motives, but they may be providing a kind of validation for her, something that she may not have experienced in her life. Even if Wanda is unaware of those feelings, they may present obstacles to looking at alternative arrangements for Carl's care. A question not addressed in the case narrative is whether there is any love between Wanda and Carl. The available information presents a very negative relationship. It would be important to know if there have been positive aspects of the relationship. As Wanda explores her own motives and feelings she may gain insight that will be helpful to her in understanding the situation and making choices.

The phone call regarding discontinuance of treatments is a worrisome event. Since Carl is terminally ill, his treatments would likely be palliative and symptomatic. A desire to discontinue these would be puzzling. One of the first goals for the physician should be to discuss this directly with Carl in a one-on-one setting. A visit should be arranged as soon as possible. Carl's current health status must be assessed and discussed and his wishes for care should be clarified. The description of Carl's status suggests that current palliative efforts are not providing much symptom relief. Medication regimens should be reviewed with attention to whether medications are being given as prescribed. Both undermedication and overmedication are of concern. Sorting out Carl's wishes for care and what has been reported might present some difficulty as discrepancies between patient and caregiver reports of events do happen. However, the discovery of this discrepancy in wishes and the knowledge that Wanda is misrepresenting Carl's treatment preferences pose grave concerns. Whether or not prior discussions of Wanda's role as a caregiver have occurred, they must happen now. The physician should explore the events that led to the phone call and discuss with Wanda the details of her current care of Carl and her frustrations. In speaking with Wanda, the physician can point out her possible options and reinforce the fact that she can make some choices. Current events can be reviewed and reflected upon to help Wanda develop insight into the need for the situation to change.

Wanda should probably not serve as Carl's sole caregiver any longer. A logical next step would be a hospice referral. Hospice could provide either in-home support or inpatient care, depending upon Carl's wishes and Wanda's interest in remaining involved in the relationship. They could assist with palliation, which would provide benefits to both Wanda and Carl. In addition, they could help Wanda in understanding the illness and its effect on Carl, so that she could distinguish between the demands of the illness and the historically unreasonable demands of Carl. This would enable her to set some limits and make decisions about what she would and would not do.

After a lifetime of victimization, the concept of making conscious life choices would present a difficult transition for Wanda and might require considerable counseling. The degree of counseling would probably exceed the scope of what Carl's physician would be able to provide. Wanda needs encouragement to explore this with her own physician and would benefit from referral for counseling with a social worker, psychologist, or other appropriate professional. However, if she could make the transition to see herself in a position to make some choices, her own frustration and anger would be lessened and she might be able to find a workable role in the caregiving relationship. It is also possible that she would choose to disengage from the relationship altogether.

An additional concern in follow up will be the delineation of a surrogate decision-maker in the event of Carl's incapacity. While that would usually be a spouse, Wanda's feelings may make it impossible for her to represent Carl's wishes. This needs to be assessed on an ongoing basis and arrangements for an alternative decision-maker might be necessary. Depending on how matters progress, legal intervention may be required.

The approach outlined above is complex and not easily accomplished. As previously noted, it would ideally have been underway prior to the events described in the case narrative. Faced with the situation described in the case the physician must now decide if these events provide sufficient suspicion of abuse to trigger a report. Carl certainly qualifies as a vulnerable adult. The issue to consider is whether Wanda is or is not providing for Carl's needs, including food, fluids, medications, and basic care. As noted previously, her unilateral decision to terminate his care is probably the major signal to the physician that there are serious problems.

The narrative also makes mention of Wanda's rough handling of Carl. The interview with Carl should include specific questions about his personal care and handling. The physician should note Wanda and Carl's relative sizes and strengths at this time, as it may not be possible physically for Wanda to provide for Carl's care. This concern can be discussed with Wanda and may provide another opening for exploring caregiving difficulties. Carl also should be examined for signs of skin breakdown or inadequate hygiene. Psychological neglect is difficult to assess in a relationship if there has never been any positive psychological support. Observations of Wanda and Carl do need to be placed in the context of the nature of Wanda and Carl's marriage.

A referral to Adult Protective Services is probably appropriate at this time. This referral should be presented to Wanda with an acknowledgement of the difficult situation she is in. The focus of this discussion should be the opportunity to provide help to Wanda in addressing her current difficulties. She should be aware, again, that reporting is mandated, but that it may lead to a better outcome than the current situation. The referral should be presented to Carl as a way of helping to provide the care he needs with recognition and reinforcement that Wanda can't provide for all of his care needs. This process may make it easier for Wanda to recognize that things must change.

The optimal solution to this dilemma would probably include a combination of hospice involvement to assist with or provide for Carl's care and help him to prepare for the end of his life, and counseling and support for Wanda. Hopefully, Wanda could make some decisions about her role in Carl's care and possibly reestablish contact with their son.

BRENDA AND HARRIET

When a frail, vulnerable older adult is providing an element of financial security for a caregiver, there is increased risk for abuse (Lachs & Pillemer, 1995; Silverman & Silverman, 2000; Kennedy, 2000). The motives of the caregiver may be less related to compassion and commitment to care and more related to self-interest. When the demands of caregiving increase, resentment and frustration build. In addition, decisions for expenditure of the older adult's financial resources may be inappropriately guided by the caregiver's financial needs. This may not occur consciously or overtly but may still occur.

When the vulnerable adult is demented, the situation becomes more complicated. A demented person may not provide any positive feedback to a caregiver. A demented person is unfortunately dehumanized more easily than someone whose cognitive and interactive abilities are intact. Finally, a demented person can be difficult or impossible to accurately interview because of the possibility of failure to remember events, lack of insight into what a caregiver is doing, and the possibility of delusional misrepresentations. Demented persons who cannot manage or even keep track of their possessions and resources may erroneously believe that family members have stolen money from them. A physician will have difficulty determining the truth of these accusations and, as a result, the accusations are likely not to be taken seriously. In the case of Harriet, for example, it might not be possible to know whether there was truth to the complaint that someone had taken her purse, or whether she was delusional or just forgetful.

The story of Brenda and Harriet states that they had been very close and suggests that Brenda loves and has compassion for Harriet. She may have assumed the responsibility of caregiver with the best of intentions. However, for a variety of reasons she is not functioning as a good caregiver for her mother.

Of the three cases presented, the case of Brenda and Harriet presents the clearest indication of elder abuse as it combines elements of inadequate attendance to safety and financial victimization. At the very least, Brenda is allowing her daughters to steal from Harriet. Harriet has problems with wandering, restlessness, and suspicious behavior. Brenda has two young children and the case narrative suggests that there are times when the children and Harriet are home alone. The children are too young to effectively care for her and cannot adequately attend to her safety. Harriet's accusations and suspicions might lead to a dangerous situation for the young children and so they also are at risk.

It is not clear whether Harriet sees a physician. Presumably, she would see someone for her chronic medical problems. Even with regular follow-up, many of the events described in the case, such as the episodes of theft, might never come to a physician's attention. As part of Harriet's ongoing care, specific questions should be asked about Harriet's symptoms at home, how she is being cared for, and what sorts of stresses Brenda is experiencing. Harriet's physician should make sure that the treatment of her chronic illnesses is optimized and that there are not untreated problems such as pain, constipation, or undiagnosed illnesses. Any of these could add to her restlessness and confusion. The circumstances of any episodes of agitation should be discussed to see if there are precipitating factors that could be improved with caregiver education. Medications should be reviewed to see if they are being accurately administered and to consider whether they may be playing a role in her behavioral disturbances. Medication also may be useful in managing mood disturbances and sleep problems, but the physician would need to watch for excessive or inappropriate requests for medication.

As noted above, Harriet's physician might be unaware of the mistreatment at home unless a crisis event, such as Harriet's getting lost and injured, were to occur. The physician would most likely remain unaware of Brenda's work-related difficulties, except for the financial difficulties faced by the family. The discussions related above might provide evidence of the difficulties in the current environment. As noted, excessive requests for medication also would be an important clue (Kennedy, 2000). Other signs of mistreatment would include missed appointments, weight loss, or frequent injuries.

Despite Harriet's dementia, her physician should attempt to talk with her alone, to see what insight she has as to the current home environment. Specific questions should be asked about how things are at home, how she's getting along, and how she spends her day. It's not clear how severe Harriet's dementia is, and her reports of events at home would need to be considered in the context of her dementia. However, if there is any consistency to her comments, they should be discussed with Brenda. It is also important to watch the interactions between Brenda and Harriet for signs of tensions and conflict. A demented person may frequently be angry with or resentful of a caregiver if that person requires someone to guide and direct them and doesn't have the insight to understand why it is happening. Consistent expressions of impatience or evidence of fear on Harriet's part are both causes for concern. The observations of how patient and caregiver interact in a setting such as a doctor's office can provide the physician with significant insight into how things go at home (Lachs & Pillemer, 1995; Kennedy, 2000).

Discussions with Brenda should include an ongoing review of the home situation, Harriet's behavior and function, and her need for supervision. The discussions need not be confrontational but carried out with an understanding of the stresses upon Brenda. However, inappropriate actions should be identified and discussed. The realization of the precarious home situation and the lack of sufficient supervision for Harriet should raise concerns and prompt discussions. Social service and nursing counseling could assist Brenda in better understanding her mother's illness and in developing strategies for caring for Harriet. Options for adult day care and respite and other resources could be explored. Referral to the Alzheimer's Association also would be helpful in providing additional education and support.

The above interventions would be useful in identifying risks for mistreatment or signs of neglect and might be useful in preventing things from getting to the point at which we now find Brenda and Harriet. However, if the physician does become aware of the safety issues and victimization, a referral to Adult Protective Services is warranted. The referral should be explained to Brenda, again as a way of helping to identify resources for help, but it is likely to be perceived as a threat, since referral could lead to placement and this would cause Brenda and her daughters to lose their home.

There are several complicating factors in this situation, the greatest of which is the dependence of Brenda and her children on Harriet for her home. In addition, it is possible that this referral may lead to another referral to Children's Services. Adding to the dilemma is the fact that Harriet might well prefer to be at home despite the problems identified. It is difficult to see a positive solution to this problem. Despite these concerns, the referral to Adult Protective Services is mandated once there is awareness of the situation at home. This doesn't necessarily mean that Harriet will be removed from the home. While investigation is ongoing, the physician and the rest of the health care team should continue to work with Brenda and Harriet, optimizing Harriet's health as above and trying to improve Brenda's understanding of the disease and its care. Brenda's health should also be assessed. Her fatigue is likely to relate to her situation, but the possibility of medical illness should be entertained. More importantly, Brenda should be evaluated for depressive illness. Counseling may be of value to her in dealing with her situation.

Although Brenda has been a victim of difficult circumstances, some of her difficulties, especially in the workplace, are apparently related to her own actions. Addressing this could be very helpful for Brenda. If Harriet remains in the home, the physician should continue to monitor for signs of neglect. The financial victimization is not something a physician could effectively monitor and might lead to the need for an outside guardian. Many of the biggest issues here are social and financial in nature. These problems will not have medical solutions.

CONCLUSIONS

The above cases illustrate some of the varied circumstances in which abuse and neglect of older adults can occur. Such circumstances may make it difficult to identify these problems, but ongoing communication and awareness can be very helpful. Suspicion of mistreatment or victimization mandates reporting. However, effective intervention requires an understanding of the context of the situations and the relationships of the persons involved. The physician should be aware of situations most likely to lead to abuse and should monitor for signs that a caregiving relationship is deteriorating or has become abusive. This effort requires the best interviewing and communication skills a physician has to offer. Ethical concerns may emerge when the patient's wishes conflict with what appears to be the patient's best interest. When this occurs, determination of decisional capacity becomes a key factor. The referral of a patient to Adult Protective Services does not end the physician's responsibility. Rather, it mandates the ongoing involvement of the physician in-patient and caregiver support and management.

REFERENCES

American Medical Association. (1992). *Diagnostic and Treatment Guidelines on Elder Abuse and Neglect.* Chicago, IL: American Medical Association.

Barbas, N.R., & Wilde, E.A. (2001). Competency issues in dementia: Medical decision making, driving and independent living. *Journal of Geriatric Psychiatry & Neurology, 14*, 199-212.

Department of Health and Human Services. (1998). The National Elder Abuse Incidence Study. Available from <*www.aoa.dhhs.gov/abuse/report/default.htm*>.

Earnst, K.S., Marson, D.C., & Harrell, L.E. (2002). Cognitive models of physicians' legal standard and personal judgments of competency in patients with Alzheimer's disease. *Journal of the American Geriatrics Society, 48*, 919-927.

Folstein, M.F., Folstein, S.E., & McHugh, P.R. (1975) Mini-mental state: A practical method for grading the cognitive state of patients for the clinician. *Journal of Psychiatric Research, 12*, 189-198.

Harrell, R.H., Toronjo, C.H., McLaughlin, J., Pavlik, V.N., Hyman, D.J., & Dyer, C.B. (2002). How geriatricians identify elder abuse and neglect. *American Journal of Medical Science, 323*, 34-38.

Kennedy, G. J. (2000). *Geriatric mental health care: A treatment guide for health professionals.* New York: Guilford Press.

Kennedy, G.J. (2002, May). Assessing the older person's capacity to remain at home: The importance of executive dysfunction. Symposium presented at the Annual Meeting of the American Geriatric Society, Washington DC.

Lachs, M.S., & Pillemer, K.A. (1995). Abuse and neglect of elderly persons. *New England Journal of Medicine, 332*, 437-443.

Lachs, M.S., Williams, C.S., O'Brien, S., Pillemer, K.A., & Charlson, M.E. (1998). The mortality of elder mistreatment. *Journal of the American Medical Association, 280*, 428-432.

Marson, D.C., Earnst, K.S., Jamil, F., Bartolucci, A., & Harrell, L.E. (2000). Consistency of physicians' legal standard and personal judgments of competency in patients with Alzheimer's disease. *Journal of the American Geriatrics Society, 48,* 911-918.

More, A.A., Seeman, T., Morgenstern, H., Beck, J.C., & Reuben, D. B. (2002). Are there differences between older persons who screen positive on the CAGE questionnaire and the short Michigan Alcoholism Screening Test-Geriatric Version? *Journal of the American Geriatrics Society, 50,* 858-862.

Ohio Revised Code. Section 5101.60-5101.62 (2000).

Rosenblatt, D., Cho, K.H., & Dorrance, P.W. (1996). Reporting mistreatment of older adults: The role of physicians. *Journal of the American Geriatrics Society, 44,* 65-70.

Royall, D.R., Cabello, M.,& Polk, M.J. (1998). Executive dyscontrol: An important factor affecting the level of care received by elderly retirees. *Journal of the American Geriatrics Society, 46,* 1519-1524.

Royall, D.R., Mahurin, R.K., & Gray, K.F. (1992). Bedside assessment of executive cognitive impairment: The Executive Interview. *Journal of the American Geriatrics Society, 40,* 1221-1226.

Schindler, B.A., Ramchandi, D., Methews, M.K., & Podell, K. (1995). Competence and the frontal lobe: The impact of executive function on decisional capacity. *Psychosomatics, 36,* 400-404.

Silverman, J., & Hudson, M.F. (2000). Elder mistreatment. A guide for medical professionals. *North Carolina Medical Journal, 61,* 291-296.

Yesavage, J.A. (2001). Geriatric Depression Scale. Available from <*www.stanford.edu/ ~yesavage/GDS.html*>.

Elder Abuse:
The Nurse's Perspective

Carol A. Miller, MSN, RN, C

SUMMARY. Nurses play pivotal roles in all aspects of elder abuse, from detection to resolution. Nurses are among the categories of mandatory reporters most frequently identified in elder abuse reporting and protective service laws, and they are the health care professionals who most often assume major responsibilities in assessing elder abuse and neglect situations. Nurses intervene in elder abuse situations as individual health care providers or as part of a multidisciplinary team. In acute and long-term care settings, nurses often work with caregivers to implement appropriate discharge plans, with the intent of eliminating risks for elder abuse. This article describes the nurse's role in addressing elder abuse, and then dramatically illustrates it with the three case studies under review. *[Article copies available for a fee from The Haworth Document Delivery Service: 1-800-HAWORTH. E-mail address: <docdelivery@haworthpress.com> Website: <http://www.HaworthPress.com> © 2005 by The Haworth Press, Inc. All rights reserved.]*

KEYWORDS. Elder abuse, role of nurses, assessment, clinical management

Nurses play pivotal roles in all aspects of elder abuse, from detection to resolution. This article summarizes the roles of nurses with respect to

---

Carol A. Miller is a Gerontological Clinical Nurse Specialist and Certified Nurse Case Manager at Care & Counseling, Miller/Wetzler Associates, and Clinical Faculty, Frances Payne Bolton School of Nursing, Case Western Reserve University.

[Haworth co-indexing entry note]: "Elder Abuse: The Nurse's Perspective." Miller, Carol A. Co-published simultaneously in *Clinical Gerontologist* (The Haworth Press, Inc.) Vol. 28, No. 1/2, 2005, pp. 105-133; and: *The Clinical Management of Elder Abuse* (ed: Georgia J. Anetzberger) The Haworth Press, Inc., 2005, pp. 105-133. Single or multiple copies of this article are available for a fee from The Haworth Document Delivery Service [1-800-HAWORTH, 9:00 a.m. - 5:00 p.m. (EST). E-mail address: docdelivery@haworthpress.com].

assessment and interventions and in relation to Adult Protective Service Law. The nursing perspective on Jane, Wanda and Carl, and Brenda and Harriett illustrates the application of these roles in three specific case scenarios. I elected to provide the nursing perspective in "first person, singular," as if I personally encountered each of the situations previously presented.

ROLE OF NURSES IN ELDER ABUSE ASSESSMENT

Elder abuse is not so much assessed as it is detected, and nurses often must assume the role of detective. Because elder abuse, by its very nature, is a hidden problem, assessment begins with a suspicion about its existence. Information may be purposefully withheld; it is rarely volunteered, except in situations in which the older person or caregiver is desperate for help. Clues to elder abuse might first be noted when an older person is seen in an emergency room or admitted to a hospital. Most often, a home visit is an essential component of the assessment process, and gaining admission to the home usually is the first assessment challenge.

Assessment of elder abuse differs from overall nursing assessment in several respects. First, in contrast to usual health care situations in which the purpose of assessment is to plan interventions for addressing health needs, the primary concern in actual or potential elder abuse situations usually is a determination of the safety of the older person. Second, health care workers dealing with elder abuse often are quite limited in their goals and they may have to accept basic safety as the only goal. Third, cases of elder abuse usually involve some element of resistance from the older person or caregiver(s). Fourth, in contrast to most health care situations, the nurse may be viewed as a threat rather than a help. Fifth, when legal interventions are being considered, the legal rights of the person and the caregivers must be addressed.

The nursing assessment of physical abuse and neglect focuses on the following aspects: nutrition, hydration, bruises and injuries, degree of frailty, and presence of pathologic conditions. When any indicators of malnutrition or dehydration are identified, the next step is to determine whether the hydration or nutritional status can be improved adequately without removing the person from the setting. Nurses can be especially important in assessing not only the nutrition and hydration status, but also the measures required to alleviate these risks immediately.

Assessment of bruises, swelling, injuries, lacerations, pressure ulcers, and other indications of physical harm is another important aspect of the detection of physical neglect or abuse. In situations of physical neglect, nurses may see any of the following indicators: leg ulcers; pressure ulcers; dependent edema; poor wound healing; burns from stoves, cigarettes, or hot water; and bruises and injuries from falls, especially repeated falls. The presence of more than one of these indicators at the same time, or over a short period of time, should raise high levels of suspicion about physical neglect. If there is evidence of injuries from falls, the nurse must consider the possibility that the person was shoved or otherwise caused to fall by someone else. Other aspects of physical neglect include substance abuse; withholding therapeutic medications; overmedicating with prescription psychoactive drugs; interfering with the person's medical care; and not providing nursing care, medical equipment, or comfort items.

Assessment of the degree of frailty of the older adult is another consideration in determining actual or potential physical abuse or neglect. In the presence of certain medical conditions (e.g., diabetes or congestive heart failure) someone may be determined to be neglected if necessary treatments cannot be or are not being provided. In determining whether an older adult can function safely in community settings, nurses consider the person's ability to follow medical regimens and the consequences of noncompliance. Assessment also addresses the question of whether the medical regimen could be modified to improve compliance while allowing the person to remain in an independent setting.

Because physical neglect can arise from the caregiver's lack of knowledge, it is essential to assess the caregiver's understanding of the dependent person's needs. Also, it is important to assess support resources, such as caregivers and friends, who influence the older person's physical and psychosocial function, either positively or detrimentally. In addition, support resources that are not currently being used are identified as potential sources of help. When the support resources currently being used are the caregivers who perpetrate the abuse, the nurse must assess the potential for working with the caregivers to alleviate the negative consequences. Although it is not always easy to work with abusive caregivers, it may be even more difficult to eliminate their influence over the older adult. During the assessment, therefore, the nurse must attempt to identify any strengths of the caregiver and any willingness to change the situation voluntarily. In assessing potential support resources, the nurse also must identify the barriers that interfere with the use of these resources.

Because a primary purpose of assessment in elder abuse situations is to determine the necessity of legal interventions when an older adult is at risk, a nursing assessment of the person's potential for safe performance of daily activities is extremely important. Personal dress, hygiene, and grooming are among the most visible aspects of daily function and people often are viewed as neglected when they do not comply with socially defined standards of cleanliness, particularly when an unpleasant odor is noted. Although poor hygiene and grooming are important reflections of many underlying problems, these aspects of daily activities do not necessarily reflect the person's safe function. Therefore, the nurse needs to assess whether the poor hygiene is hazardous to the person's health. She also needs to assess the consequences of imposing assistance with personal care on someone who may be unwilling to accept help or to acknowledge a hygiene problem. Adequate nutrition and hydration, and an ability to obtain help in an emergency, are the basic human needs that are most often called into question in cases of elder abuse. Other basic needs also may be compromised, usually in relation to specific functional impairments and environmental circumstances. For instance, for people who are bed-bound or who have very limited function, bowel and bladder elimination may be a basic need. For people with mobility limitations or serious vision impairments, safe ambulation and the ability to avoid falls are important considerations.

Nurses also assess the immediate living conditions to determine whether minimal standards of safety and cleanliness are being maintained. For example, nurses evaluate the person's ability to maneuver in the environment during daily activities, as well as the person's safety in emergency situations, such as a fire. Likewise nurses examine the neighborhood environment for its impact on the safety of the person. This is especially important when the older person lives in an area of high crime or extreme isolation and is vulnerable by virtue of impaired judgment, physical frailty, or a combination of physical and psychosocial impairments.

In assessing potential neglect situations, nurses consider the potential influence of seasonal conditions that are likely to increase the risk for elders who live in climates characterized by extreme heat or cold. For example, a person who does not pay utility bills may not be in any danger as long as the weather is mild, but when the temperature turns cold, that person would be at risk for hypothermia. The same is true for people who occasionally wander outside without dressing appropriately. As long as the neighborhood is safe and the weather mild, they may be relatively safe; however, they may be at increased risk during the cold months, especially if they do not wear proper foot covering.

The most immediate consideration in determining whether legal interventions are necessary is the assessment of threats to life. In home settings, it is frequently the nurse who assesses the urgency of the situation and whose opinion is used as the basis of legal interventions. Situations often are viewed as being of crisis proportions when they are first discovered, and the immediate reaction of the person who discovers the situation may be to remove a person from the environment. Many times, however, the person may not want to leave the home setting, or there may be no better setting in which the person can receive care immediately. In these situations, the nurse may be asked to assess the urgency and seriousness of the situation and to provide an opinion about whether or not legal interventions are justified. The nurse often is viewed as the person who can either convince the elder to accept help or convince the caregivers and social workers that the present situation is tolerable. At times, nurses are successful at convincing the person to accept help, especially if they assure the person that, with proper help, the situation can be improved.

In situations in which the caregiver is the abuser, the nurse and other team members must assess whether the caregiver presents a threat to the life of the dependent older person. If there is any evidence or history of physical violence on the part of the caregiver, and if the dependent elder does not have the ability to escape or otherwise defend himself or herself, a threat to life may exist. Threats to life also may exist if serious medical conditions are untreated or inadequately treated. The nurse may be the health professional, especially in home situations, whose opinion is essential in determining the consequences of action or inaction. Lastly, suicide potential must be assessed, especially for self-neglected elders who also are depressed and expressing feelings of hopelessness.

In cases of elder abuse, the nurse often plays a major role in assessing the person's capacity for reasonable judgments about self-care. When judgment is impaired to the point that the person is at serious risk and does not acknowledge the risk, the person usually is considered incompetent or incapacitated. The crucial element in assessing the risk for elder abuse, therefore, is a determination not of the goodness or wisdom of decision-making abilities, but of the danger, if any, posed by the decisions. When the competence of an older adult to make safe decisions regarding self-care is in doubt, nurses may be legally bound to make reports or consider other legal interventions.

ROLE OF NURSES IN ELDER ABUSE INTERVENTIONS

Elder abuse is one of the most complex and challenging situations that nurses encounter, because it usually is a compilation of many problems involving the older person, the caregivers, and the environment. The focus of nursing interventions vary according to the setting in which nurses work. In acute and long-term care settings nurses can intervene in cases of elder abuse through their work with caregivers and their participation in discharge planning. When elder abuse is rooted in the caregiver's lack of information about adequate caregiving measures, the nurse can teach the caregiver about the person's care before discharge. In addition, when nurses are concerned about a caregiver's abilities, they can initiate a referral to a home care agency or a public nursing agency for follow-up. In some cases, the nurse may ascertain that the situation requires skilled nursing care, covered by Medicare, for at least a few visits. If the nurse has serious questions about a discharge plan that seems inadequate, a referral to a protective service agency may be made so that the situation can be monitored on a long-term basis.

Caregivers of dependent older adults who are temporarily in institutional settings often seek advice from nurses about the management of the dependent person's care. They may be ambivalent about taking the person home, or they may be unsure or unrealistic about their own ability to provide appropriate care or to cope with the stress of the situation. In some cases, the caregivers may be seeking permission not to provide care at home, and they may seek this permission in indirect ways. In these situations, nurses often are in the best position to facilitate communication among all the decision makers, including the primary care provider, the older adult, and the various family members who are responsible for care. When nurses identify caregiver concerns, they can suggest individual counseling or support groups. One of the most effective ways to prevent elder abuse is to provide support and education for the caregivers, and the best opportunities for this may arise when the dependent older adult is in an acute or long-term care setting. Nurses can encourage caregivers to use the period of institutionalization to reevaluate their own abilities to provide care at home, as well as their own need to accept additional support and assistance.

Nurses in home settings have many opportunities for teaching caregivers about adequate care through verbal and written instruction. In addition to teaching caregivers directly about the provision of physical care and the management of difficult behaviors, nurses and home health aides also can serve as role models. Some caregivers may have great difficulty managing complex medication regimens; in such cases, the nurse can simplify these regimens through the use of charts and specially designed plastic containers. Nurses also can educate caregivers about basic care needs, such as nutrition, exercise, and elimination. In working with homebound people, nurses may need to identify essential resources for an initial medical evaluation or for ongoing monitoring.

Nurses in home care agencies play important roles in working with home health aides and other caregivers, both in recognizing and intervening in situations of elder abuse. Home care nurses must educate home health aides about the detection of elder abuse, and they should be available if home health aides have questions or concerns about what they observe. If the home situation cannot be discussed openly during supervisory visits, the nurse may have to arrange a time for private discussion with the home health aide. In situations in which the older adult requires a significant degree of physical care or supervision, the services of a home health aide may be the most effective means of preventing elder abuse. Often, however, the retention of a home health aide in such difficult situations depends largely on the degree of support and guidance provided by a professional nurse.

Nurses in other community settings, such as clinics or senior centers, also have opportunities to intervene in elder abuse. In these settings, nurses often come in contact with spouses who have assumed a caregiving role and who need advice about resources to assist with the care of the dependent spouse. In addition, nurses will encounter older people who neglect themselves and need support services at home. Older adults and their caregivers may not be aware of the many community-based services that are available, and the nurse may be the only professional with whom they have any contact. Community-based resources, such as congregate meal programs, home-delivered meals, or adult day care centers, may be an effective way of preventing or alleviating some situations of elder abuse or neglect. Nurses can facilitate referrals for whatever services are appropriate.

In home and other community settings, the nurse is usually the professional best positioned to identify the need for health services and facilitate appropriate referrals. Moreover, with the growing demand for home care services, there is increased availability of diagnostic tests that can be performed in the home (e.g., radiographs, blood tests, and electrocardiograms). In many situations, these diagnostic tests are essential for determining whether involuntary care measures are justified. For instance, if the older adult refuses to go out of the home for care, home-based diagnostic measures may provide the evidence needed to convince the person or the primary caregiver that hospitalization is warranted. On the other hand, results of these diagnostic tests also may be used to convince caregivers, protective services workers, and involved professionals that hospitalization is unnecessary.

Nurses can facilitate referrals for services that will decrease the burden of caregiving responsibilities and improve the older adult's self-esteem and level of independence. For instance, speech, physical, and occupational therapy may be useful in improving the older person's ability to communicate, ambulate, and perform daily activities. Nurses also can suggest medical equipment and assistive devices that would improve the person's function and relieve some of the caregiver's responsibilities. Caregivers may be unaware of disposable supplies and the many assistive devices that are available, and they may be quite responsive to suggestions from the nurse about obtaining and using these items. Any interventions that improve unsafe situations may prevent or alleviate elder abuse or neglect.

Finally, services aimed at reducing caregiver stress or dealing with caregiver problems also may prevent or alleviate elder abuse. Mental health counseling or support groups may be quite helpful when abuse is related to caregiver stress. Respite services can be provided through in-home care, by companions or home health aides, or through the participation of the dependent older person in adult day centers. Sometimes, even a limited amount of respite will be sufficient to prevent or alleviate elder abuse in situations in which the caregiver is stressed and overburdened.

NURSES AND ADULT PROTECTIVE SERVICE LAWS

As health care professionals, nurses are among the categories of mandatory reporters most frequently identified in elder abuse reporting and protective service laws (Tatara, 1995). This is appropriate because the various duties ordinarily assumed by nurses place them in a critical position for witnessing the consequences of abuse and neglect. In addition, a primary role of nurses is to foster collaboration between health care professionals as abuse reporters and adult protective service or law enforcement officials as abuse investigators or service providers.

Protective service workers frequently call upon nurses to assess older people suffering from abuse or neglect. Indeed, nurses frequently are the preferred health care worker for conducting such assessments owing to their holistic approach to health assessment, their availability through public health departments or visiting nurse associations, their willingness to make home visits, and the relative ease with which older people usually accept them. Nurses provide essential care and treatment for abused and neglected older people. They help correct the conditions caused by maltreatment and self-neglect, and they prevent their recurrence through such activities as treating injuries, monitoring medication, educating caregivers, obtaining assistive devices, and facilitating service referrals.

In addition to assuming primary roles in assessment of and interventions for abuse or neglect, nurses frequently serve as consultants to protective services workers when questions arise regarding the health status of clients. Typical questions relate to medications, continence, nutrition and hydration, and disease signs. Another consultant role for nurses is to train adult protective service workers in health assessment, disease identification and detection, recognition of endangerment, and other topics. Occasionally, nurses assume roles in submitting records and providing testimony in the cases of elder abuse that are referred to courts. In all their roles, nurses work cooperatively with other professionals and with paraprofessionals, applying their expertise and experience in an attempt to help elders who are abused or neglected.

NURSING PERSPECTIVE ON JANE

Initial Nursing Visit (Monday, the Day After Jane's Visit to the Urgicare Center)

As the visiting nurse who saw Jane last winter, I had orders from the doctor at the Urgicare Center to visit three times a week for dressing changes. When I knocked on Jane's door for my initial visit, she yelled for me to come in. She was sitting on the couch, which was near the remains of the burnt chair. A fire was burning in the fireplace, which had no screen in front of it. There was an ample supply of wood next to the fireplace, and a stack of old newspapers in front of it. She apologized for not getting up and said "I'm just too slow with my old Arthur bones." Jane was wearing a dirty terry cloth robe and frayed and worn out slippers that were much too large for her feet. I suspected that the slippers originally belonged to someone else. Her hair was matted and disheveled and I noticed that her feet and ankles were swollen. Her eyes were a little bloodshot. A glass half-filled with a dark liquid sat on the table next to her. I thought I detected a smell of urine, but with the fire burning and all the other odors it was hard to tell. When I tried to get close enough to smell her breath, I thought that maybe it had an alcohol-sweet aroma–again, it was hard to tell what I smelled.

Four cats checked me out from the other room, and I guessed that there were at least 4 more around the house. Initially the clutter, the smell of cat litter, and the environment that seemed very bleak to me took me aback. I had worked in this rural county for ten years, and I had seen a variety of situations and met hundreds of people who had grown up in this area, so I wasn't concerned about Jane's isolation. She was like so many others who preferred solitude. What did concern me, however, were the dearth of groceries on hand and her seeming unawareness of the need to plan for getting more food and other supplies. Luckily, I carried all the supplies that were necessary to change the dressings on both her hands, but I knew she wouldn't be able to drive until her hands healed and I wondered how she would get food for her and the cats. The supply of food in her house consisted of an open box of powdered milk, about 5 boxes of macaroni and cheese, and a limited number of canned goods (mostly soups, a couple cans of corn, some tuna fish, and corned beef hash). She told me she had plenty of food in her cupboards, but I had sneaked a peek in her cupboards when I was in the kitchen washing my hands and she couldn't see me from the living room. I estimated that her food could last for no more than a week. In addition to the food, there were 6 bottles of apricot brandy in the cupboard. I also checked the supply of cat food and kitty litter and estimated that the 2 bags of dry food wouldn't last more than a week if I was accurate in guessing that there were about 8 cats in the house. The bag of kitty litter was almost empty, but she didn't seem to use very much of that at a time. At the very most, the cat food would last for 2 weeks, and I suspected that Jane would be more concerned about the supply of cat food–and apricot brandy–than she would be about her own supply of food.

I wasn't sure if what I assessed as her "unawareness" arose from lack of insight, her long-term pattern of privacy, or from her staunch spirit of self-sufficiency. I was sure she'd be upset if she knew I looked in her cupboards, so I needed to use this information cautiously. Jane told me that a neighbor from a few miles away came by at least weekly to see if she needs any groceries. When I inquired about the neighbor's name, she said "She just goes by the name of 'Sally.'" When I inquired about what day of the week Sally comes, she said "Oh, I never know. It's whenever she happens by this neck of the woods." I observed that Jane did not have any calendars visible and the only clock I could see was in the kitchen. When I asked questions as my subtle way of assessing

Jane's mental status, she was very vague or she answered with another question for me. For example, when I asked her if she knew what day of the week it was, she said "What's the matter with you? Don't you know? Why do you have to ask me? Get yourself a calendar if you need to ask that kind of question." She set clear limits on answers to any of my questions, so I was reluctant to ask about much.

When I was changing the dressings on Jane's hands, I asked how she was managing to get the usual things done, like getting washed, going to the bathroom, and preparing food. She said she is managing just fine, but she's a little slow because of her arthritis ("old Arthur"). She refused to show me how she walked or managed any of her other activities of daily living and cut off my questions by saying "Sally will come by if I need anything." She told me that Sally didn't have a phone so she couldn't give me any number for her. Sally's address was simply "the farmhouse up the road a bit." At one point during my visit, Jane stated "You ask too many questions. It's too bad you need to come back because you're a bit nosey for my liking."

Thoughts After My First Visit

I need a better assessment of Jane's mental status, but I sure don't know how I'll get it. I suspect she has some dementia that she's trying desperately to cover up, but I could be wrong. I also suspect she was drinking apricot brandy right before my visit, but she's entitled to enjoy whatever she wants, since she's not diabetic as far as I know. Of course, she hasn't had any medical care for years, except what was done yesterday at the Urgicare Center, so maybe she does have some medical problems. I doubt that they did any blood tests. Her feet and ankles were swollen, but mine would be, too, if the only thing I ate was canned foods. I was afraid to suggest a homemaker or meals-on-wheels, since she was adamant about Sally taking care of whatever she needs. I suspect that "Sally" exists only in Jane's mind, but I'm not sure how I'll ever find that out. I thought about offering to open a couple cans of food, but then she'd know I snooped in her cupboards; besides, she'd tell me that Sally would be stopping by soon. I don't think she'll be able to use that old-fashioned can opener with the bandages on her hands. The referral from the Urgicare Center indicated that she is supposed to see a burn specialist for follow-up in a week. She insisted that she'll call the number on the paper and Sally will take her, so I can't say much more about that to her. I wonder if she can use the telephone? I think she's the one who called 911 when she had the fire, so I guess she can use it OK.

I noticed a couple of fire hazards, but I'm not sure how I can approach her on that. There's no screen in front of the fireplace, and she keeps a stack of newspapers right near the open fireplace. She already had one fire that I know about, and who knows if there's been other fires. She doesn't have any smoke detectors, but she told me that she asked Sally to get her one. I sure have a hard time fighting Sally's help! I don't think she moves much from in front of the fire place, so she's likely to notice if there's a fire–at least if she's awake and alert enough. On the other hand, her judgment and awareness seem impaired, so she's more likely to be burnt and not be able to get help. I think I'll ask my supervisor if our agency can dip into our "Cookie Jar Fund" and buy her a screen for her fireplace. I've used that fund for other worthy causes and that would be a good way to resolve this safety hazard. I can call the fire department and ask them to come by with a smoke detector. They installed one for another patient when I called them last year. They know about the fire in Jane's house, because they came to put it out and took her to the Urgicare Center. I'll ask them not to tell her that I called; they can just tell her that they do this routinely after a fire. Maybe they'll check around for other fire hazards and talk to her about some safety issues. I do worry that Jane can't move very fast to get away from a fire. At least she keeps her phone next to her and I know she can call 911. It's too bad the phone cord stretches across the pathway between the living room and the kitchen. Maybe she'll let me rearrange the cord so it's not a fall hazard.

I need to develop a plan for getting more food in the house, because it will be a month before her hands healed enough for the bandages to be off and she certainly can't drive with those bandages on. Of course, I can't challenge her information about Sally too much, and I doubt that she cares much about whether or not she has food. I'll try to capitalize on my suspicion that she'd at least worry about getting a supply of cat food and kitty litter. I'm glad that she appreciates the use of kitty litter, even if she is a little stingy with it. By next week, she's likely to let me arrange for grocery shopping, because she'll be out of cat food. I suspect she'll also worry about getting some more apricot brandy, but I'm not going to bring up that subject–she can bring it up herself.

Third Visit (Friday After the Visit to the Urgicare Center)

This is the third time I've visited Jane, and she is sitting on the couch. She looks pretty much the same as she did the last two times I came. When I peek in the kitchen cupboards I notice that a few of the cans are missing and there's only 3 bottles of apricot brandy today. Jane reports that Sally has stopped by twice this week. She also reports that she has an appointment with the burn specialist next Tuesday and, of course, Sally will take her. She emphasizes that Sally has been a great help and she's glad she can count on her. After my last visit, Jane removed the bandages from the fingers on her right hand, and today she refuses to let me put bandages on any of her fingers. I tell her that I need to put dressing on all her fingers and both hands because that's what the doctor ordered. When she sees the burn doctor next Tuesday she can ask him about not having so many bandages. She again assures me that Sally is planning on going to the grocery store tomorrow and "you needn't mind my business about food–do I look like I'm starving?"

Thoughts After My Third Visit

If anyone had been to see Jane since my last visit, there would have been tracks in the snow, and there are none. I suspect that I've been the only visitor all week. I think Sally is a figment of Jane's imagination and she serves a very useful purpose when I ask questions. I'm not sure how I can challenge this or get to the bottom of her reality. I suspect that Jane will have the dressings off when I come on Monday, because this is the only way she can manage to use the can opener. I again offered meals-on-wheels, but she told me that Sally was coming by to help. I think it's enough of a breakthrough for her to let me in when I come; she's not likely to accept a homemaker or meals-on-wheels. When I ask questions, she still gives vague answers. She's actually quite clever in her responses; I can tell she's an educated woman. Based on my assessment during these three visits, I'm pretty sure that Jane is in the early stage of dementia. But, maybe she has some medical problems that are causing the cognitive impairment, or maybe the apricot brandy is the problem. Whatever is going on, I wish I could get her assessed, because I hate to overlook anything that's treatable.

Someone as private and independent as Jane would do best if she can stay in her own home, but if her mental status is impaired, she would be at risk staying there alone. If she is in early stage of dementia, she could be taking something like Excelon and she could probably stay in her own home a lot longer. Before Execelon and the other anti-dementia drugs were available, it was easier for me to ignore the early-dementia people because there wasn't any treatment anyway. Now I have a different dilemma–I feel obligated to try and get them the treatment that might keep them more independent. Sometimes, I wish we didn't even have these options, because then I wouldn't have as much responsibility to try to get a good medical evaluation and find out if the person has dementia. Of course, with her drinking so much alcohol, that's likely to be at least a contributing factor, and she's not likely to agree to stop that. I think her apricot brandy is more of a friend to her than Sally is. Perhaps it's best to just let her and the brandy live their life with those cats. It does bother me, though, that I might be overlooking something treatable. If I ignore this situation, it's certain to deteriorate and she's sure to end up back at the Urgicare Center. Even worse, she might have a serious problem and not even get any help.

I think I'll contact the burn doctor that she's seeing on Tuesday and find out if he will suggest that she go to Dr. J. M., because he has been so good with a couple of my other patients who have needed a good assessment. If I could get Jane to see Dr. J. M., at least he would check for medical problems and maybe I can get him to do a mini-mental status assessment so I have some idea of what's going on. Maybe Dr. J. M. would get a blood alcohol level if I asked about that. I also could ask him to check for diabetes, hypothyroid, and vitamin deficiencies. I bet Jane has some medical problem and maybe she'd take a pill if it meant that she could be more independent and stay in her own home. It would be easier for me if she would admit that there's something wrong. Maybe I can break through her denial and defensiveness. I think I'll try to be friendlier with her cats and then maybe she'll talk to me more.

I noticed that there's a smoke detector in the living room; I was pleased that the fire department had followed through with helping me out on this one. This might be backfiring though, because when I said I was glad to see it, she smugly said "See, I told you Sally would be coming by and she brought the smoke detector just like I told you she would." Now it will be all the harder to challenge Sally's existence; I don't want to let her know that I had asked the fire department to install the smoke detector. Besides, if I challenge Sally's existence, that will ruin the fragile relationship I have with Jane. When I told her that I was bringing a fireplace screen that I had been storing in my basement, she said "Well, I guess I'll have two of them then, because Sally's going to bring one next week. If you want to get rid of some trash from your basement, that's OK with me." At least I'm making some progress on the safety issues.

Fifth Nursing Visit (Wednesday, Ten Days After the Visit to the Urgicare Center)

As usual, Jane is sitting on the couch. I bring the fireplace screen with me–I removed all the labels and added a little dirt so it doesn't look brand new–and put it in front of the burning fire. I ask Jane if I can move the stack of papers off to the side, and I'm glad that she doesn't resist. She tells me that the screen that Sally is getting for her will be a lot nicer, but "I'll keep your basement trash for now if it'll make you happy." I tell her that it will make me very happy. The bandages have been removed from her fingers since my last visit, and I ask her how her appointment with the burn specialist was yesterday. She says that Sally had car trouble, so she rescheduled the appointment for next week. I'm relieved that her burns are healing despite the fact that she takes the dressings off soon after I leave.

I ask her about the names of her cats and she rattles off about 7 names. Despite my allergies, I extend my hands to the friendliest of the cats and I try to befriend one of them. I engage her in extended conversation about the cats, and I work my way up to asking about whether she'll be needing food for the cats. I know the supply is dangerously low, because I checked the cupboard again and there's only a small amount of dry food. My nose tells me that the kitty litter has run low–or out. She relies on her usual Sally response, and I gather up enough courage to say "If Sally is having car problems, she might not be reliable enough–I'm sure you want to be certain that you've got enough food for all these wonderful four-legged friends of yours." My strategy isn't entirely successful, but she admits "If you come by before Sally gets here again, I guess you can bring the cats some food." When I suggest that I could get the county senior companion program to send someone to do the grocery shopping, she adamantly says "You can bring some cat food if you've got some stored in your basement, but don't you be sending no do-gooder to help me when I don't need any help. Sally's car is going to be fixed tomorrow. I told you to keep out of my business."

Thoughts After My Fifth Visit

I'm disappointed that Jane didn't go to the burn doctor, because the nurse in his office promised me that they'd try to get Jane to go see Dr. J. M. If Jane doesn't keep her appointment with the burn doctor and she's not compliant with keeping the dressings on, then she won't qualify for skilled care visits from my agency anymore–at least she's still homebound. I suspect that she'll begin to drive if there's no other way to get cat food and apricot brandy, and I wonder how safe she is driving. The nearest store is 9 miles away. Even if I got her some groceries and cat food, she'll need the brandy, and even the county worker might not get that for her. My supervisor approved of buying the fireplace screen from our Cookie Jar Fund, but I doubt that she'll approve of more expenditures and I'm sure not going to ask about buying brandy for Jane. I wish I could get a better assessment of Jane's mental status. The more I talk with her, the more convinced I am that she's got some dementia. It's very likely that she also has some medical problems, because her feet and ankles are still swollen.

At least I've made some progress with the safety issues, but I still don't know if she can make any phone calls, except for 911. I guess if she can call 911, then she's safe enough. I finally moved that phone cord from the pathway, but there's still all those extension cords that don't look very safe to me. I'd like to see the bedroom and bathroom to check for hazards, but she's sure to accuse me of being too snoopy–she's already accused me of being snoopy and she doesn't even know I've peeked in her cupboards. If I push her too far, I'm sure she'll have the door locked the next time I come. I can see that she'll never accept any homemaker for the grocery shopping–besides, if I make a referral to the county companion program, the homemaker would want to clean up the kitchen and that would be the end of the homemaker service as far as Jane was concerned.

Seventh Visit (Monday, Two Weeks After the Initial Visit)

As soon as I pull up to Jane's house, I notice that her car has been moved and there are fresh tracks in the snow. She is seated on the couch as usual and calls for me to come in. She looks pretty much the same as she usually does, except there are no bandages on her hands. She tells me she won't be needing me again because her hands are all better. I examine her hands and assess that the burns are mostly healed, but there are some deep scabs and reddened areas. She does not have full range of motion for her fingers and it looks like some of the burn wounds could still get infected–she also could get contractures where all the scar tissue is forming. She has been using the cream that was prescribed at the Urgicare Center and she insists that she doesn't need any help with anything. I check the cupboards when I am in the kitchen and I find 8 bottles of apricot brandy, a supply of cat food, and several cans of soup. Jane tells me that Sally stopped by and went to the grocery store for her. Sally will be taking her to the doctor appointment tomorrow, and there's no need for me to come back. Jane is going to start keeping the door locked, because she's seen some suspicious foot prints in the snow. She's not going to let anyone in anymore–"including Miss Snoopy Nurse, even though you're a very nice person."

Thoughts After My Last Visit

I guess Jane is pretty self-sufficient. Even if she'd let me back in, Medicare wouldn't pay for the visit, because she's not compliant and she's not even homebound anymore. She's got what she needs to survive. I've addressed some of the safety concerns, but I sure do wonder about her mental status, especially her ability to make safe decisions. I also worry about her driving and hope she's safe enough out on the roads–and that other people are safe with her out on the roads. I know that Jane's cognitively impaired, and I suspect that there's at least one medical intervention that could be done to improve her functioning, but I don't think she'd cooperate with any treatment–especially if it involved giving up her brandy. But, on the other hand, shouldn't she have the benefit of an assessment, so a professional could talk to her about her choices? Maybe if she understood that giving up brandy and getting treatment for medical conditions would improve her functioning and enable her to live independently she'd choose to cooperate. I know that independence and staying in her own home are extremely important to her. If I make a referral to Adult Protective Services, perhaps they can get her to agree to an assessment.

Supervisor's Analysis of the Nurse's Assessment and Interventions

The visiting nurse had a lot of barriers to deal with in establishing a relationship with Jane, who for so many years led a reclusive lifestyle. If she hadn't used some good techniques, she would never have been able to visit five times. She did not challenge Jane's statements about Sally, even though there's good reason to believe that Sally does not exist. Also, even though the visiting nurse is allergic to cats, she was friendly toward them and used them as a topic of conversation so Jane would accept her a little more. The visiting nurse was astute in her observations and she used subtle questions to assess Jane's mental status. She also did a good job of identifying some major safety concerns and finding creative ways of addressing fire hazards, fall hazards, and other safety risks. Even though sneaking a look in Jane's cupboards might seem like a violation of privacy rights, it was important to find out if Jane had enough food for survival. By the third visit, the visiting nurse began filling out our agency abuse/neglect assessment form and this was helpful when it came time to refer the case to Adult Protective Services.

Ethical dilemmas that the visiting nurse dealt with included issues of freedom over safety and the right to personal choices and decisions. Because she was able to resolve the major safety issues in Jane's house, Jane's level of risk was reduced and the visiting nurse could respect Jane's choice of living arrangements. She also had concerns about Jane's driving and potential risk to the safety of others, and these concerns were not directly addressed. The visiting nurse included a statement about her concerns in the referral to Adult Protective Services and requested that they address this issue. Her other ethical dilemma was related to a professional obligation to identify health problems that could be treated, while respecting Jane's right to refuse treatment. The visiting nurse had good reason to believe that Jane had some treatable conditions and that Jane's health, functioning, and ability to remain in her own home would improve if these conditions were addressed. At a minimum, Jane should have an opportunity to make an informed decision about the potential effects of her choices. The visiting nurse was clever in her attempt to arrange a referral for an assessment, but these efforts were not successful. To resolve this dilemma, she referred Jane to Adult Protective Services with the expectation that a comprehensive assessment would be done.

NURSING PERSPECTIVE ON WANDA AND CARL

Observations from the Initial Nursing Visits

As the hospice visiting nurse, I made my initial visit based on the referral by Carl's doctor and the unenthusiastic permission given by Wanda when I called to arrange for my visit. During the course of my first four visits, Wanda has confided about their many years of unhappy marriage and I now know more about their relationship than I ever wanted to know. I repeatedly set limits on the time I spend with Wanda, because she takes me aside as I'm trying to leave and she says she needs to talk about Carl. She usually begins the conversation by focusing on how bad Carl is getting, but then she spends most of the time talking about how hard it is for her to take care of him. When I suggest that a home health aide be assigned to help with the care, Wanda insists that Carl would never let anyone except her do anything for him. She insists that it would be a waste of anyone else's time, because he would make sure Wanda did all his care before the home health aide came. When I've assessed Carl, he has been polite but extremely impatient and demanding—I suspect that he is on his best behavior for my benefit and I hope that I never see his worst behavior. He confirmed that he would refuse to have anyone but Wanda do his care; he told me the only reason he lets me come is because his doctor insists on getting reports from a nurse before he calls in refills on the pain medications–if he didn't need pain medication, he would "fire the whole lot of you."

Thoughts After My First Four Visits

My relationship with Carl is pretty tenuous and I'm not sure that I can establish any effective relationship with Wanda. My impression so far is that this is a long-term unhealthy marriage–at least by my standards–and they are not requesting marital therapy from me (and even if they wanted it, I'm certainly not qualified to provide that service). I always have a hard time dealing with women who stay in abusive relationships for years on end–I don't understand why they just don't leave. Whenever I have to deal with these situations as a visiting nurse, I have to put a lot of effort into being nonjudgmental–it's not easy for me to have empathy for these passive women. Carl refuses any interventions except pain medication and Wanda would like some relief from the situation, but she's dug her own hole by allowing him to dominate her life all these years–how can I possibly have any impact?

I think a home health aide would be helpful in alleviating some stress for Wanda, but I don't see any way of getting Carl to accept that help– even if he did accept the home health aide, he's likely to be verbally abusive toward the aide and I'll have to spend a lot of time mending fences and trying to make this plan successful. With my caseload, I can't spend that much time just to get a home health aide established in a situation where there's such resistance. Besides, Wanda has chosen to live in this kind of relationship with Carl for all her adult life and who am I to try to change it? On the other hand, maybe Carl is not mentally competent anymore and certainly he needs a lot of care because of his cancer. If Wanda can't–or doesn't–provide the care, shouldn't I insist that a home health aide help? I suspect that Wanda doesn't give him much fluids and he may even get dehydrated. I've noticed that he seemed pretty confused when I visited him this week–perhaps that's because he's dehydrated. It also might be because of his cancer, but with him refusing to see the doctor, I don't have good information about his medical status. Even if I had more information, I'm not sure what I could do about it–I'm not in any position to change this situation. Maybe I should just discharge the case as noncompliant. I guess I should discuss it with my supervisor.

Advice from the Nursing Supervisor

As the nursing supervisor for the hospice nurse, I understand the pressure she is under to prioritize her cases and not spend too much time on those that aren't very cooperative or receptive to care. However, the hospice program was established to address the needs of dying patients, and certainly this is a needy situation. The hospice nurse needs to think of this situation as a potential Adult Protective Services case–she says a referral is not warranted because this is just a long-standing abusive marriage, and Wanda has been perfectly capable of making informed choices. The hospice nurse assumes that because Wanda has chosen to stay with Carl for all these years, she is competent to make her own choices and we should respect these choices without interfering. However, I am concerned that Carl has become more abusive and demanding–certainly his care needs are more demanding–and the pressure on Wanda is significantly greater than it used to be. With this mounting pressure, Wanda may be less competent to make decisions than she used to be. On the other hand, the hospice nurse, says that Wanda is less at risk than she used to be, because Carl no longer has the strength or ability to be physically abusive. Wanda also is in control of his care now, and she can decide whether he gets food, drink, medications, and other things he needs.

Perhaps a report needs to be made on Carl, because I suspect that his physical needs are not being met and he may be at risk of dehydration, and who knows what else. I also wonder if Wanda is withholding Carl's pain medications in retaliation for how he treated her in the past. The hospice nurse needs to consider whether Wanda is competent to make good decisions about Carl at this time. She also needs to consider that Carl's verbal and psychological abuse of Wanda might meet criteria for elder abuse, even though it's not a new problem. The hospice nurse might be obligated to report both the abuse of Wanda by Carl and the neglect of Carl by Wanda.

I agree about not pushing for a home health aide, at least at this time. Although an aide would likely assure that Carl gets better care–at least while the aide is there–I doubt that Carl would accept the help and he would likely be abusive to her. Besides, Wanda would still be in charge of Carl's care for the rest of the time, and care from the home health aide would be just a drop in the bucket, so to speak, in relation to all his needs. It's too bad that Carl can't see that a home health aide might provide better care than Wanda, but he has such control issues, it's not likely that he would have that perspective. I don't think he's figured out that Wanda is gaining control over his situation because he is dependent on her for all his physical needs now. He's very adamant about not wanting more people coming to the house–probably he doesn't want anyone else to see what their situation is. The hospice nurse is right about her perception that we'd have to spend a lot of time working with the situation before placement of a home health aide would be successful, and we just don't have that kind of time to invest in a hopeless situation. I'll advise her to visit a couple more times and see what she can find out about Carl's mental status–as well as Wanda's ability to make appropriate decisions. We need more assessment information so we can determine if a referral to Adult Protective Services is warranted. The hospice nurse needs to do some more research on identifying suspected verbal and psychological abuse of Wanda and neglect or even maltreatment of Carl. I'll ask her to begin using the agency elder abuse and neglect assessment form so we can document any decisions. In fact, she needs to fill one out for each of them. If we don't make a referral and a crisis develops, we need to be able to defend our decision and that assessment form will be helpful for whichever direction this case goes. As much as she doesn't like Carl's attitudes and behaviors, the hospice nurse needs to establish more of a relationship with him, so she can do a better assessment of his needs and his possible willingness to accept any outside help.

Thoughts and Observations from the Next Four Visits

I've visited Carl and Wanda weekly for another month and I've been successful in getting him to talk with me for 15 minutes at a time. He's not so cranky with me anymore, except when I suggest that I could arrange for a home health aide to come. After the discussion with my supervisor, I decided that I could establish a better relationship with Carl by asking him about his son. Of course, I know from Wanda that the son is estranged, but Carl still likes to talk about him and he wants me to think they have a good relationship. After I got Carl talking about his son, I was able to find out a little more about the care Carl gets from Wanda. He says Wanda is "good enough" about leaving water for him and he's learned not to drink too much at a time, so one glass of water will last all day. However, when he asks for any juice or food, she usually waits about an hour before she brings it. He insists that it doesn't matter much because he's never very hungry anyway. I have been weighing him when I visit and he's been losing about a pound a week for the past 2 months. Every time I visit, Carl says he's having severe pain–8 on a scale of 1 to 10–but Wanda tells him she can't give him any medication because it's not time yet. Carl told me that the doctor said he could have pain medications every 4 to 6 hours if he needed them, but Wanda told him that the doctor changed the order to one pill no more than every 8 hours. Wanda says the doctor didn't order enough pills for him to take it more than every 8 hours, so she can't give it to him whenever he demands it. Carl says he never talks to the doctor, because the phone is downstairs and Wanda makes all the calls. When I called the doctor to clarify the orders, I found out that the pills could be taken every 4 hours if needed. However, when I counted the pills in the bottle, only half the expected number was there. I sure do wonder if Wanda is taking some of the pills for herself–or maybe she's just squirreling them away for another time.

Wanda continues to take me aside for long discussions about Carl, but I have managed to set limits on how long she talks by telling her as soon as I walk in that I have to leave in an hour. I also told her that I need to hear more about Carl's care and less about their marriage. I know I need to report to my supervisor about my assessment of Wanda, so I try to focus on how she's coping with Carl's care. It's no surprise that she expresses a lot of anger toward him, and makes statements such as "He's finally getting what he deserves after all these years." She's always vague when I ask her to explain that kind of statement, but I suspect that at least one of the things she thinks he "deserves" is to suffer some physical pain without getting the pain medications as prescribed. I try to get Wanda to talk about the emotional impact of Carl's illness on her because I'd like to get a better idea of her stress, but I'm not very successful in getting her to answer any of my questions about this.

I'm still hoping that we can get a home health aide in the situation and I know I need both Carl's and Wanda's cooperation on that. I've made some progress in getting Carl to see that if a home health aide was there, then he might get his pain medications more frequently and he also would have more control over his meals and other care needs. Now I need to get Wanda to see that a home health aide would provide some relief for her and allow her some time to go out, at least to the store. She's been leaving Carl alone when she goes out for a couple hours at a time, and he doesn't even have a phone near his bed. I made some progress in getting Wanda to agree to get a portable phone so Carl would be able to call for help when he is alone. Wanda hasn't gotten the phone yet, but she promised that she would. I don't think it's a good idea for Carl to be alone, but if he could make a phone call, then the risk would be minimal and that would be acceptable. Based on some of the things

Wanda has said, I think she hopes something will happen to Carl when she's gone, and she wouldn't care if he could get help or not.

Advice from the Nursing Supervisor

I reviewed the agency elder abuse and neglect assessment form that the hospice nurse filled out for each of them. Clearly, there is some evidence of Wanda withholding medications from Carl–this would suggest the need to report to Adult Protective Services. The nursing assessment of Wanda does not show enough evidence of psychological or verbal abuse to warrant a referral of her at this time. The hospice nurse reports that Wanda no longer complains so much about Carl, although she suspects that when nobody is around Carl's behaviors are quite difficult, if not outright abusive. Somehow, though, it doesn't seem fair to refer Carl because Wanda withholds medications, when Carl's the one who has been abusive for so many years. A referral to Adult Protective Services at this time would make Wanda look bad, and she's the one who's been suffering for many years. Also, if the hospice nurse makes a report to Adult Protective Services now, Wanda and Carl are sure to figure out that she's the one who made the report and that will ruin any relationship that she has established with them. Furthermore, I think that our hospice agency will do a better job than Adult Protective Services in working with this situation. I'll advise the nurse to monitor the situation for a while longer and see what develops. Perhaps her interventions will resolve the neglect aspect of this situation. I'll also get our social worker involved in counseling Wanda–I think if Wanda had someone to confide in about her own issues, then she might develop more appropriate ways of handling her anger toward Carl. Our social worker is good with these situations and we could justify coverage for her services under hospice, because Wanda's behaviors directly affect Carl's health. Perhaps if we could get the home health aide in there, that would relieve some of the stress on Wanda and it would also give us more information about the care that Carl receives. Most importantly, it would give us control over at least some of Carl's care and we would know that he is getting food, fluids, and medications appropriately.

Thoughts and Observations from the Next Visits

I finally got Carl to agree to try a home health aide by suggesting that he would get his pain medications every four hours as needed if a home health aide was there every day. Even though the aide can't give the pills, she can follow the schedule that I set up and she can make sure his pills are available for him. I'm relieved that Wanda let me set Carl's pills out in a daily dose container–I told her that the doctor had ordered me to do it that way, because it was important that I be able to give accurate reports to the doctor about how much pain Carl is experiencing and I can do a better assessment if I know how much pain medication he needs. I also was able to teach Wanda about the benefits of giving the pain medications on a regular basis rather than waiting until Carl's pain got so bad that he couldn't stand it. I convinced Wanda that if Carl had his pills more regularly, then he would be in a better mood and would be more cooperative. Wanda seems to go along with my suggestions–even though I suspect there are some secondary gains for Wanda from seeing him in pain.

Because Wanda now confides in the social worker, some of her needs are being addressed. Wanda has a lot of built-up anger to deal with and the social worker has helped her develop some better coping mechanisms. If she can deal more appropriately with her anger, then Carl is more likely to get better care. I hope Wanda follows through with our suggestion that she attend the support group for spouses sponsored by our hospice program. I arranged for the home health aide to be scheduled at the time the support group meets so Carl wouldn't be left alone. We've had a home health aide assigned to Carl for four hours daily and he seems to be more comfortable.

Initially I had to spend a lot of time smoothing the ruffled feathers of the home health aide when Carl yells at her, but she's pretty tolerant by now. I've been able to get Carl to behave a little more appropriately by telling him that the aide is very sensitive and that his shouting scares her. Also, I set up a simple room monitor system so Carl can have some privacy and be alone sometimes, but the aide can hear him when he calls. The two-way monitor system enables the aide to verbally respond immediately even when she is downstairs. I think some of Carl's cantankerousness was because he was scared of being alone so much and afraid that Wanda would never come with his food or pills. Now that he knows that the aide will be there when he needs something, he seems a lot better and less demanding. Those inexpensive room monitor systems have been a big help for a lot of my patients and they are so easy to find in baby supply departments.

Thoughts of the Nursing Supervisor

The hospice nurse has made a lot of progress with Wanda and Carl. After getting over the initial hurdles–including her own difficulties with having to work with a long-term unhealthy marriage situation and her inclination to feel empathy primarily for Wanda–she established effective relationships with both of them. By getting the home health aide and social worker involved, she was able to address a lot of the issues and avoid a referral to Adult Protective Services–at least for the time being. I know that she will closely monitor the situation and continue to assess the need for a referral. I agree with her that the risks have been minimized and both Carl's and Wanda's needs are being addressed by hospice. It's likely though that as Carl's condition worsens–which it will–the stress will mount again and additional interventions will be necessary. However, if we can maintain our current plan, we'll have a good head start on dealing with problems that develop in the future.

NURSING PERSPECTIVE ON BRENDA AND HARRIET

Observations During the First Visit

As the county health nurse, I received a referral from the emergency department after Harriet was brought in. The doctor suspected that this is not the first time that Harriet has been wandering the streets not knowing where she is or how to get home–it's just the first time that she's been brought to the hospital. I think the hospital should have just referred Harriet right to Adult Protective Services, but they made the referral to us because our agency has an agreement to send a public health nurse out to do a follow-up assessment on any older adults who seem to be at risk and come to the emergency department but aren't admitted.

My initial visit was with Brenda and Harriet, and they were both very cordial. Harriet's mental status is obviously impaired and she was quite repetitive during most of my visit. She must have told me about her purse at least 50 times. Harriet wanted to focus the entire conversation on all the money she is missing and she tried to convince me that Brenda has been taking all her money. Brenda kept cutting her mother off and telling her that her money is in the bank and they couldn't get it until the bank opened in the morning. Harriet got quite agitated when Brenda repeatedly told her they couldn't go to the bank until tomorrow; at one point Harriet raised her hand to hit Brenda, but Brenda moved out of her way and Harriet hit the table instead. After that, Brenda suggested that Harriet watch her favorite television program, and I was able to talk with Brenda alone while Harriet stayed in the den where the television was. I know that people with dementia often get fixated on money–women inevitably talk about purses incessantly–but I have to wonder if Brenda does dip into her mother's money. Of course, she certainly deserves compensation for taking care of her mother, so I expect she would use her mother's money.

Initially, Brenda stated that her mother is "a piece of cake compared to what I do with 14 wacky people all day." She said her mother had been diagnosed with Alzheimer's disease several years ago and has had diabetes and high blood pressure for about 10 years. She's supposed to take two "high blood" pills and one pill "for her sugar" every day, but the pills are "pretty costly." Sometimes Brenda cuts them in half, especially at the end of the month, so they can be stretched out. Brenda makes sure that her mother gets at least one whole "high blood" pill every day and if she gets only a half of the "sugar" pill Brenda makes sure she doesn't eat any candy or sweets that day. Harriet used to check her own blood sugar regularly, but she forgot how to use the glucometer and Brenda is too busy to bother. Besides, those test strips are expensive.

Brenda takes her mother to the doctor about once a year because that's the only way she can get the medications refilled. When I looked at the dates on the medication bottles, I noticed that the last refill for 30 pills was two months ago and that all the pills in the bottle were cut in half. When I estimated the number of pills left in the bottles, I concluded that Harriet is lucky if she gets half the prescribed pills. The emergency department report stated that Harriet's blood pressure was 178/102; when I checked it during my visit, it was 156/98. Brenda says she plans to take her mother for an annual doctor appointment next month. She promises me she will ask the doctor about Harriet's diabetes and blood pressure at that time.

When I asked Brenda what is the hardest part of caring for her mother, she broke down in tears and talked about how hard it is when Harriet gets upset with Brenda's children and tells Brenda that her daughters have stolen all her money. Sometimes when Brenda comes home from work, her daughters are outside playing and they refuse to spend time with their grandmother because they say she is so mean to them. Brenda has seen bruises on her mother's arms, but her daughters always explain that their grandmother bumped into a chair or wall while Brenda wasn't there. Brenda denies that she keeps her mother locked up at times, but I noticed a sliding lock on the outside of both the front and back doors. It looks to me like these locks are used when the family wants Harriet to stay inside and they want to be outside. There's a deadbolt on both doors, also, and they can use that from the inside. Brenda says that she has been advised not to leave her mother alone, so she never does. I suspect that Brenda's daughters are not very concerned about leaving Harriet alone and I'm convinced that Harriet spends long periods alone on a regular basis. I ask Brenda if she is aware of the "Safe Return" program sponsored by the Alzheimer's Association for people who are at risk for wandering. Brenda says, "They told me about that in the emergency department, but I'm sure it costs a lot of money and it would be a waste because we never leave her alone anyway."

Based on the assumption that Harriet is alone at least some of the time–even though Brenda denies this–I assess safety issues that might be pertinent. When I ask about the gas stove and oven, Brenda says that her mother once turned it on and left the burner on without flames, but Brenda smelled the gas and nothing happened. That was about six months ago, and Brenda is sure that her mother has forgotten how to use the stove so she's no longer worried about that. Besides, there's a sign on the stove that says "out of order" and she thinks that will keep her mother from using it. I notice that there are no smoke detectors in the kitchen, or anywhere else in the house. Brenda says she bought a couple about a month ago, but has been too busy to put them up.

When I ask if Harriet could make a phone call if she needed help, Brenda says "Probably not, but there's no need for her to use the phone. She can just shout for one of us, because we never leave her alone." When I ask about meal preparation, Brenda reports that her daughters get cereal and milk for Harriet, and there's always plenty of food in the refrigerator–"They all just help themselves and they do a fine job–the food keeps disappearing, so they must be eating it." When I talked with Harriet earlier in my visit, I noticed that her clothes were pretty large for her, but Brenda denies that Harriet has lost any weight and she says, "She's always been pretty skinny."

Thoughts After My First Visit

I'm sure that Harriet is left alone and isn't safe, and I suspect that there may be some physical abuse of Harriet. It also seems pretty clear that Harriet doesn't get her medications for diabetes and hypertension as ordered. It's likely that her blood sugar is high and that would certainly compromise her mental functioning even more than it is with the dementia. In addition to not wanting to spend the money on test strips for the glucometer, Brenda probably doesn't want to know what her mother's blood sugar is, because it's likely to be high and Brenda would feel obligated to give her the correct medication. Being a nurse's aide, Brenda knows the implications, but I'm sure the dominant influence is that she doesn't want to spend more money on medications. There are ways of dealing with the cost of medications–perhaps the doctor could prescribe less expensive medications (I noticed that the pills were not generic), or Harriet could get her prescriptions through one of the medication assistance programs offered by most of the drug companies. Of course, Brenda would have to put some time into arranging for that and she's not likely to make the effort–it's so much easier for her just to deprive her mother of the pills.

Brenda is at the point of burn out, but she is so resistant to having help, because she'd have to use some of Harriet's limited assets. If Harriet went to adult day care, she would be safe and she would get at least two good meals a day. If Brenda understood the importance of controlling her mother's diabetes and hypertension so her mental functioning would be better, maybe she would be more reliable in making sure her mother got appropriate treatment. If I make a referral to Adult Protective Services at this point, Brenda will be angry with me and I won't be able to teach her about her mother's medical conditions. I'll plan one more visit and hope that she pays attention to my advice.

Observations During the Second Visit–Two Weeks After the First

I check Harriet's blood pressure and it is still high: 168/104. When I have Harriet take her sweater off so I can check her blood pressure, I notice bruises on both upper arms. I can tell by the different colorations of the bruises that they have occurred at different times. When I ask Brenda about the bruises, she said "I told you last week we had a big problem with her walking into chairs and walls–we can't keep track of her all the time and we can't get rid of all our chairs just so she's safe."

I bring a glucometer, and Harriet's blood sugar an hour after lunch is 204. I talk with Brenda and emphasize that high or low blood sugar has a direct effect on mental functioning and high blood pressure is a major risk factor for small strokes that can cause dementia. Brenda seems to understand my points, but she says that her mother's had both problems for so long it can't make much difference. Besides, the medications are too expensive and her mother doesn't like to take them anyway. A friend told her about those medication assistance programs, but the friend said a lot of paperwork and phone calls are involved in getting the pills and she certainly doesn't have time to bother. Besides, Brenda sees "lots of people at the nursing home who have sugar and high blood and they're no wackier than the others." Brenda tells me I'm making too much of her mother having Alzheimer's disease and "she gets along a lot better than all those I take care of all day at the nursing home." I make a referral to Adult Protective Services for further assessment.

REFERENCE

Tatara, T. (1995, May). *An analysis of state laws addressing elder abuse, neglect, and exploitation.* Washington, DC: National Center on Elder Abuse.

Elder Abuse:
The Social Worker's Perspective

Carol Dayton, MSW, ACSW

SUMMARY. The role of social work, and specifically Adult Protective Services, is described in three case studies. Intervention in the lives of older adults and their caregivers is presented through the social work skills of psychosocial assessment, relationship building, and empowerment. Information and opportunities are presented to the older adults under analysis in order to maximize independence and control over decisions that affect their daily lives. In each case the critical issue of an allegation of harm is investigated by Adult Protective Services, including the potential impact of a range of legal interventions. *[Article copies available for a fee from The Haworth Document Delivery Service: 1-800-HAWORTH. E-mail address: <docdelivery@haworthpress.com> Website: <http://www.HaworthPress.com> © 2005 by The Haworth Press, Inc. All rights reserved.]*

KEYWORDS. Elder abuse, adult protective services, role of social work, clinical management

THE ROLE OF SOCIAL WORK

In responding to the three case studies under discussion, the analysis in this section is not only specific to the profession of social work but to

Carol Dayton is affiliated with Cuyahoga County Department of Senior and Adult Services, Cleveland, Ohio.

[Haworth co-indexing entry note]: "Elder Abuse: The Social Worker's Perspective." Dayton, Carol. Co-published simultaneously in *Clinical Gerontologist* (The Haworth Press, Inc.) Vol. 28, No. 1/2, 2005, pp. 135-155; and: *The Clinical Management of Elder Abuse* (ed: Georgia J. Anetzberger) The Haworth Press, Inc., 2005, pp. 135-155. Single or multiple copies of this article are available for a fee from The Haworth Document Delivery Service [1-800-HAWORTH, 9:00 a.m. - 5:00 p.m. (EST). E-mail address: docdelivery@haworthpress.com].

135

the interventions that would occur were a report regarding these circumstances received by the Adult Protective Services (APS) staff at the Department of Senior and Adult Services in Cuyahoga County, Ohio. This public agency (located in Cleveland) is the legally mandated recipient of all reports alleging abuse, neglect, self-neglect, and/or exploitation of community-dwelling impaired adults age 60 and over residing in the county, as is each of the county human service departments throughout the state for older adults in their locales. A social work response reflects the commitment of that profession to accept individuals as they are, enhancing the dignity and worth of the person, assessing psychosocial functioning and the environment, using an approach based on identified strengths, including the available support system. The social worker perspective considers opportunities and choices that respect self-determination and maximize the independence of the client. As well stated by Nelson, Eller, Streets, and Morse (1995), older adults will be seen as complete in themselves, and the social worker will honor them as survivors. Supporting, enabling, and empowering older adult clients are the key goals in adult services, usually requiring collaborating with other systems, since the problems rarely fall in simple or singular categories.

The decision whether or not to make a report to APS Intake is a common experience in the extensive network of agencies and professionals assisting the elderly. That decision focuses on the assessment of impairments, physical and/or mental, as well as the indicators of suspected harm. It is the combination of these two factors that necessitates a report to APS.

Due to the intersection of social work and law that is represented by APS, the clients are non-voluntary, characterized by the fact that the individual and the staff have no alternative to the legally mandated face-to-face contact that must be made for the purpose of investigation. Even though the nature of work is with non-voluntary clients, the social worker will continue to strive to affirm the dignity and worth of each individual, a particular skill and strategy described by Rooney (1992). For purposes of this discussion, the assumption is that from any number of possible professional sources, concerned citizens, or involved parties, a report has been made to APS and the case is being considered for investigation. It is unlikely for these three individuals, or the older adult population in general, that the older adult will directly request assistance from APS, accusing a family caregiver of inflicting harm or being neglectful. Rather, the client will more typically be protective of the caregiver out of shame and/or fear of a negative outcome, or due to diminished capacity even to recognize the harm that is occurring.

Each of these three case studies are discussed with the same beginning event, a call to the APS Intake staff (a call unknown to the older adult). The discussions also include the likelihood and nature of any other social work interventions by aging, legal, or health care service providers.

JANE

This case presents a typical situation of an intentionally isolated individual who is determined to manage independently and is successfully doing so until physical and/or emotional decline escalates the risk of harm to the point of detection. It is likely that Jane's circumstances were called into APS twice, and this discussion will examine the likely outcome of the APS investigation in each instance.

The first report received by APS most likely would have been made by the visiting nurse one year prior to the present set of difficulties being experienced by Jane. The nurse arrived to care for the burns on her hands and by doing so was the only other person to enter the house in over twenty years. The characteristics of self-neglect would have been evident: a furnace that has not been repaired for approximately nine years with a resulting fire risk of dependence on a fireplace as the sole source of heat; excessive clutter increasing the risk of a devastating fire; risks now complicated by the physical impairments of diminishing vision and increasing arthritis; likely poor personal hygiene as a result of the necessity of layers of unchanged clothing in order to remain warm; and an apparent refusal to consider any change in these conditions to reduce future risks of injury or death. Jane's lack of interest in improving her conditions or reducing her isolation may well have conveyed depression to the visiting nurse, whose primary focus is short-term and limited to changing the dressing on Jane's burned hand.

The visiting nurse is a mandated reporter to Adult Protective Services and identified as such in Ohio law (Ohio Revised Code 5101.61). The questions to be addressed in the telephone interview between the nurse and the APS Intake social worker are (1) whether the individual is sufficiently impaired physically and/or mentally to be unable to provide for self-care and protection, and (2) whether the conditions of self-neglect exist (in this instance, the issue of neglect by caregiver is not relevant). In Ohio law, self-neglect is the failure of an adult to provide the goods or services necessary to avoid physical harm, mental anguish or mental illness to self. The circumstances of the burn indicate impairments. The chronic and deteriorating conditions of poor vision and arthritis contributed to the accident, and the continuance of these hazardous conditions without any interest in improving them indicate the failure to provide adequately for self to avoid harm. The description also would have raised some alarm about the issues of mental anguish and mental illness in relation to possible depression and/or dementia. The nurse may have suspected the alcoholism as well. On the basis of these conditions, an investigation by an APS social worker would occur in response to the call from the visiting nurse one year prior to the winter storm being described in the case study.

Self-neglect accounted for 51.9% of the allegations of harm received by APS in Cuyahoga County in calendar year 2001. This is a somewhat lower percentage than the overall rate in Ohio. Self-neglect is a difficult phenomenon to define and is not uniformly identified in APS statutes across the country, with every state having its own unique statement in law in regard to adult protective services. The literature regarding self-neglect identifies it as an area needing further research in regard to its extent and nature (Gruman, Stern, & Caro, 1997). The article describes a research study that compared self-neglecting older people and other victims of elder abuse in the state of North Dakota. The findings of this study indicated that self-neglecting older adults are more likely to be living alone, socially isolated, and displaying physical impairment, mental illness, alcohol/drug abuse, and psychiatric impairment when compared to victims of abuse.

The APS social work investigation and assessment of Jane would start no later than three days after the report by the nurse was received, including the first visit to the home. This three-day time line to start the investigation is specified in Ohio law, with the exception being a life-threatening emergency when the investigation must begin in no more than twenty-four hours. Investigation timelines vary by state. During the thirty day investigation of Jane the social worker would call the nurse to inquire regarding details and any further updates. In addition, the nurse would receive a letter from the Chief of APS indicating the names and telephone numbers of the assigned social worker and supervisor should further contacts be needed. The identity of the referral source is not revealed to the client or other concerned individuals. However, in Jane's case and in many others, the client often will make an assumption regarding the identity of the reporter, conveying resentment and anger at the uninvited arrival of a government social worker. Following contact by the social worker, Jane may have considered as possible sources of the referral (1) the staff of the urgent care center, based perhaps on her layered clothing and the story of the fire, even though they do not directly know the conditions of her home; (2) the nurse who has now seen what others have not; and (3) "meddling" neighbors, aware of a small fire at the home of an eccentric elderly woman living alone. In response to even the most astute guess, the APS social worker must maintain the policy of not discussing the referral source at all. The underlying belief is that revealing or confirming such information may jeopardize any ongoing efforts of the referral source to be of assistance, as well as creating a disincentive to making future reports.

It is likely that Jane would have refused admission of the APS social worker to her home, maintaining that she is "fine," that the nurse is attending to her needs, and that the accident was a one-time issue that should not prompt any further concerns. Jane is likely to display anger and agitation at receiving the written notice of explanation of the purpose of the investigation, a formal notification described in the APS law (ORC 5101.62). The notice is given on the first visit and is a statement of the purpose of the initial interview, explaining that a call has been received by APS indicating that the individual may have been abused, neglected, or exploited, or may be unable to take care of his/her own needs. The statement also indicates to the client that help may be needed to protect the individual or his/her interests, and that it is the responsibility of the county department to investigate the report to determine if the person is safe and receiving adequate care, and to offer services based on that assessment. In addition, the social worker explains that the interview is to determine if help from APS is needed or not, and not to make accusations or prejudge any situation. Gaining access to the home of the reluctant and non-voluntary client is often an obstacle. Based on the assigned social worker's individual judgment of how to initiate the investigation, a telephone call to arrange the interview may have been made. The case study does not indicate if Jane has a telephone; her entrenched isolation indicates this is unlikely. However, if a telephone is available, it is likely Jane will attempt to prevent an arranged appointment, only to learn that the home visit is in fact a requirement of APS law (ORC 5101.62).

The initial interview is important in establishing the purpose of the investigation as well as the presentation of a helping relationship by the APS social worker. Regarding Jane, the critical question is her mental status and capacity to understand her risks, make decisions regarding those risks, and carry out her decisions. Based on what is known from the case study, it appears that Jane's mental status concerns are current and with recent onset, including confusion (becoming lost when a detour required learning new information), and not being able to recall recent and routine events (forgetting breakfast). It is not likely these indicators of decline would have been significant enough to be detected a year earlier. Jane's aloofness and eccentricity have been longstanding lifestyle issues that had not caused previous risks of physical harm.

This first entry of APS into her life is likely to have been brief, not welcomed, and quickly leading to her articulate and insistent refusal to consider changes in her dwelling that would improve her safety by repairing/replacing the furnace. Cost and inconvenience are the reasons Jane would present to explain her refusal to change. Less obvious would have been the symptoms of her depression and unresolved grief, leading to difficulty with concentration and decision-making, an inability to view the future as a time to plan for, not just a time to endure.

The APS social worker would consult with the doctor who treated Jane at the urgent care center and also with the visiting nurse regarding their clinical impressions of her mental status. The APS assessment instrument also requires a functional assessment of Jane's mental status and decision-making capacity, as well as the risks and supports in her environment. There are no indications in the case study description of the time period when the burn occurred that significant mental impairments were present. The outcome of the APS intervention would be to confirm that a physically impaired woman is self-neglecting in regard to the safety of her dwelling, is mentally clear and alert and comprehends her risks, and has refused the recommendations of the APS social worker to assist her in utilizing the various low-interest and no-interest loans for senior citizens to make home repairs. One additional referral is likely to be discussed with Jane, referral to a local senior center/nutrition site for socialization and information about senior citizen benefits and activities. If this referral is acceptable to Jane, the agency social worker or outreach worker would be contacted by APS to make a visit to encourage her participation, since Jane is highly unlikely to initiate any contact on her own. However, even if a successful referral were completed and a visit made by the agency social worker, Jane's lack of receptiveness to new relationships and resistance to intrusions into her privacy are likely to prevent a successful and ongoing contact.

Based on review of these activities and approval of the APS supervisor, the case would be closed. As in many APS cases, the social worker will experience the uncertainties involved in closing a case when an individual both remains at risk of serious harm and has the mental clarity to refuse offers of assistance and has done so. The social worker must resolve an internal struggle over the lack of satisfaction with such an outcome, as well as the understanding that the person's right to self-determination has been honored, a value held high by the social work profession. Jane and the involved parties (nurse and possibly the local senior center staff and the doctor if they had ongoing follow-up contacts) are notified of that decision and an offer of future help extended if anyone involved believes that further investigation by APS was needed.

The principles that guide APS practice offer an ethical and legal underpinning to what are difficult choices in determining appropriate interventions. The ethical struggle to respond in the best interest of the older adult is particularly difficult when a mentally clear and alert adult is at risk of serious harm and even death. The autonomy-paternalism dilemma in social work has been considered a critical issue in the delivery of services to the elderly (Abramson,1985).

The critical principles that guide the APS response to the referrals regarding Jane are listed in hierarchical importance (Anetzberger, 1988):

> Freedom Over Safety: The client has a right to choose to live at risk of harm, providing he/she is capable of making that choice, harms no one and commits no crime.

> Self-Determination: The client has a right to personal choices and decisions until such time that he/she delegates or the court grants the responsibility to someone else.

> Participate in Decision-Making: The client has a right to receive information to make informed decisions and to participate in all decision-making affecting his/her circumstances to the extent that he/she is able.

> Least Restrictive Alternative: The client has a right to service alternatives that maximize choice and minimize lifestyle disruption.

The discussion of each of the case studies will refer to the most critical principles, those above as well as others. In cases such as Jane's where the community is eager for a problem to be solved ("they consider the house and the land eyesores"), it is helpful and common for the principles to be a source of explanation and understanding.

Bringing this case discussion to the present moment, the occasion of the severe storm, the impassable condition of the roads and the dwindling supply of food, it is now a quite different sequence of events. Winter storms draw communities to the level of caring that can be undetectable on an ordinary day. The second contact with APS Intake may be based on a call from a concerned citizen, asking the county sheriff to go to Jane's home because they also are unable to risk driving on the roads and suspect that their eccentric and difficult elderly neighbor may be out of food and firewood. The local grocer who knows the exact pattern of Jane's grocery needs may seek the sheriff's assistance in checking on the absent customer who is likely to be out of food and not able to risk traveling. The sheriff department deputies check on Jane, find her confused, experiencing vision and ambulation problems that create life-threatening risks in her handling of the fireplace, and nearly out of food. They insist on taking Jane to the local senior center, where food, warmth, and companionship are being provided for the isolated elders at risk during the storm. Jane resists, argues, her confusion increases, but the deputies prevail and drive Jane to the center. Safety forces are mandated reporters to APS and believe Jane is an impaired woman in need of protection from her own limitations and the harm that can result from self-neglect. They also call APS, describe her living arrangements, agitation and confusion, and their concerns regarding her return home once the storm subsides.

The sheriff's call to APS Intake is reviewed for the issues of impairment and allegation of harm, and the case is then assigned to the same social worker that met Jane a year ago. This continuity is important in assessing any changes in functioning over time, but also can be helpful in establishing more quickly a pattern of intervention and offer of help for the client. Jane is visited in her home, having returned there when the storm abated and the roads were cleared. The storm and relocation have increased her agitation and disorientation. She is struggling to again present herself as able to control her own affairs as she had a year earlier. Self-control and preserving one's own identity are often key issues for isolated older adults in situations that present problems of self-neglect. Strategies for responding to self-neglect cases emphasize recognizing the strong attachment to objects and places. Minimizing disruption and taking time to develop some rapport are valuable practices in responding to a self-neglect case when the crisis is not immediate (Bozinovski, 1995). The social worker recognizes that Jane has declined in her mental and physical functioning in the last year, that the assessment will require a thorough geropsychiatric evaluation; to accomplish this, winning Jane's cooperation will be valuable. Jane has had a frightening experience in increased dependency during the storm and, fortunately, is open to her new visitor, the social worker.

It is at this point that a more detailed history-taking occurs, including some beginning understanding of Jane's profound grief at the loss of her partner. Her depression has lingered and deepened without an appropriate outlet due to Jane's long ago established secrecy about her life as a lesbian. The complex issue of self-neglect by lesbian and gay male elders is considered by Cook-Daniels (1997) in her examination of four key issues: internalized homophobia, history of hiding, the value of independence, and the fear of encountering homophobia.

Jane's rejection of outsiders and her longstanding isolation from peers and neighbors convey the likelihood of the key struggle underlying these issues is the effort to define oneself as worthy and decent in the face of strong negative social prejudice. This central issue is nearly inevitable for lesbians or gay males of Jane's generation, having lived throughout their adolescent and adult years in a society that normalized prejudice in regard to sexual orientation. A key adaptive outcome of this experience is to cultivate and hold tightly onto one's independence, creating the difficulty presented by Jane in accepting any outside intrusions. The APS social worker must listen carefully for the impact and meaning of the relationship with Jane's "house mate"/partner without intruding beyond Jane's point of comfort. Eventually, it will become apparent that the intensity of the unresolved grief and longstanding isolation from positive social supports has complicated and made more critical the mental health/mental status evaluation that is being planned.

As discussed by Peach, Koob, and Kraus (2001), loss of significant relationships and the subsequent grief are often associated with a diagnosis of progressive dementia and are poorly understood. Grief often contributes to depression. Jane's use of alcohol also is now disclosed and understood by Jane and the social worker to be a response to this history of isolation and loss and a contributing factor to her decline. The APS social worker receives assistance from the department's behavioral health nurse in assessing Jane and discussing with her the critical importance of having a thorough examination to understand her increasing forgetfulness and confusion. Jane agrees and an in-patient assessment is arranged.

The APS social worker is relieved that the legal option of a civil commitment order for a mental health evaluation is not necessary. Jane's voluntary acceptance of an evaluation stems from her own fears and the acceptance and support of the social worker. Without that agreement, the social worker would have consulted with the supervisor and the Probate Court Psychiatric Unit regarding the appropriateness of a mental health order for removal to a psychiatric facility for evaluation on the basis of apparent depression and dementia combined with the high risk of a fire. The provision for this involuntary admission is described under the mental health section of Ohio law (ORC 5122.01). When utilized, the individual who has been deemed a danger to self or others is removed by police, usually a traumatic event in itself.

The remaining steps in the APS intervention for Jane will be determined by the evaluation. If in fact there is significant dementia, a guardian may be necessary to make decisions in Jane's best interests, ideally based on an understanding of her life values and preferences. The social worker is hopeful that treatment of the depression, substance abuse counseling and follow-up, and a subsequent agreement by a more emotionally stable and mentally alert client to begin fixing up the house and repairing the furnace will make Jane's independence and return home possible. After all, the cats give her the experience of being needed. The house contains the history of the love relationship that gave meaning to her for much of her adult life.

However, if Jane refuses treatment and any improvements in the safety of her home, the case must be reviewed with APS legal counsel regarding whether legal interventions and court-ordered protective services can be justified. The Ohio Protective Services for Adults Law allows for petitions to be presented to the Probate Court by staff of the department of human services (or appropriately designated agencies) for the purpose of obtaining an order authorizing the provision of protective services that have been refused by the incapacitated individual at risk of harm (ORC 5101.65).

The question will be the degree of Jane's incapacity to make reasonable decisions in regard to her basic needs and the degree of risk to her safety. The Court examines carefully the facts presented by APS and Jane herself and/or her legal counsel to determine if removal of the adult's right to make independent decisions can be justified, even for the brief fourteen day period established in APS law. If the conditions warrant a Protective Service Order and involuntary removal to safety by the police force, the APS social worker would seek the least restrictive environment for Jane, perhaps a group home or assisted living if her care needs do not justify nursing home care. The termination of the time-limited court-ordered services requires again the consideration of guardianship and a surrogate decision-maker if Jane's decline warranted such an extreme intervention at that time. Probate Court will contact next-of-kin identified by APS to inform them of the pending legal decisions.

Throughout this series of possible legal actions there are the practical considerations that are always present and require social worker attention: Who will care for the cats? (Considerable time can be used in locating an appropriate source of public or private shelter/care until a final legal action is taken and the question of a decision-maker settled.) Who will close up the house and secure it, if needed? (Probably the sheriff will undertake this task, if Jane is removed against her will.)

Ongoing review of this case will continue until there is a more stable situation or a medical and legal determination of Jane's ability to make her own decisions. If it is determined that Jane can make her own decisions, a series of referrals would be offered, including mental health and substance abuse counseling through private agency resources, as well as the array of senior citizen resources for meals, socialization, home repair, and group support for older gays and lesbians through a local community resource center. Long-term case management will be considered for Jane if she is willing to accept the ongoing involvement of social service providers. This could be provided by either the county or private agencies, depending on Jane's preferences and service availability. If Jane is found upon medical evaluation unable to make her own decisions and a guardian is appointed, the recommendations for services will be presented to the guardian who is likely to be an attorney selected by the court, since Jane has assets, at least to the extent her house and savings provide.

Jane's story illustrates well the dilemma discussed by Longres (1994), "where does self-determination end and self-neglect begin?"

WANDA AND CARL

One of the difficulties in this case is establishing distinctions between the victims of harm and the perpetrators of harm in the present situation. The roles of abused and abuser have blurred over time, as the dynamics of power and control have shifted. The longstanding tension regarding Carl's physical and emotional abuse of Wanda has now come to the point of role reversal, with Wanda using her husband's illness and dependency as an opportunity for retaliation. It is unclear in the case description but likely that the present situation includes continuing verbal and emotional abuse of Wanda by Carl.

One scenario in this case analysis is that Carl's physician telephoned APS Intake to discuss his concerns about the recent call he received from Wanda stating the decision to cancel treatment. He is likely to be reluctant to bring in a government authority to examine the concerns he has regarding the case, wanting to respect the privacy of his patient who is terminally ill and to maintain his exclusive authority over the dynamics of the care plan. However, the call to cancel the cancer treatments was disturbing. Since the doctor has known Carl, he has been an opinionated and demanding man, not one to let his wife make decisions or even communicate decisions made by him. The doctor has suspected for a long time that the marriage is poor and the wife's care is only what is required. Her anger and bitterness have been increasingly evident. The doctor now suspects that Wanda is not only neglecting her husband's care but that she may be handling him roughly when she does respond to his requests. Also, he suspects that Wanda has taken over the decision-making of a still competent man without his knowledge or consent. However, it is not hard for the doctor to have both an understanding of Wanda's reactions and some level of sympathy. After all, he suspects that Carl has been terrible to her. There seems to be deep bitterness toward each other and significant harm to Carl could be the result. The physician recognizes his duty as a mandated reporter to APS and reluctantly calls Intake.

One of the first issues that APS Intake staff will address is the question of who is the client in the context of the APS investigation. There is no question that Carl is severely impaired physically; however, Wanda has no stated impairments, a requirement in Ohio law to be considered a vulnerable adult appropriate for protective services (a component of APS law that varies widely from state to state). Carl is presented as needing protection from Wanda in regard to her alleged neglect of his care needs, loss of emotional control in regard to her rough handling of him physically, and violation of his rights by making critical care decisions without his participation or consent. While Wanda has suffered longstanding abuse from her husband, and may still be the victim of the verbal and emotional abuse he has heaped on her over the years, her lack of impairments precludes a case from being opened that would focus on her need to be protected from further abuse.

The focus of the APS involvement with Wanda will be on the allegations regarding her care of Carl. Her need for help as a victim of domestic violence can be addressed through referral to the providers of domestic violence programs in the community, with the objective to find an appropriate support group for older victims of longstanding abuse. It is likely that the Intake social worker will consult with the Intake supervisor about the discomfort of identifying Wanda as the alleged perpetrator of harm, recognizing from the description her longstanding experience of being a victim.

If Carl were receiving hospice services due to his terminal diagnosis, counseling by a social worker would be available to both Carl and Wanda. Is it likely that the history of anger and violence by Carl would be openly revealed to the social worker? Wanda's poor self-esteem and history of social isolation, and Carl's deteriorated physical condition, make it unlikely that they would self-report. However, the presence of Wanda's anger and deep bitterness could provide sufficient reason to inquire and offer both an opportunity to examine the past and address the present issues regarding Wanda's care of Carl and his approaching death. This period of time is in fact a last chance to address issues that have long been held silent in this battering relationship. It may even be the first "safe" chance to do so from Wanda's point of view. For hospice staff, it is also likely that Wanda's sudden decision to end Carl's treatment would lead to a report to APS, if in fact a report had not been made earlier based on the questionable care.

Brandl and Raymond (1997) have examined the dynamics of older battered women. Their analysis of the issues has led to careful distinctions regarding the origins of the abusive behavior. The plan for intervention must carefully identify whether the harm is the result of the limited capacity of the caregiver, the stress of caregiving, or a domestic violence pattern of coercive control that one person exercises over another. The characteristics of domestic violence include inflicting physical harm, instilling fear, and preventing victims from doing what they wish or forcing behavior that is not wanted or chosen. Abusers inflict deliberate suffering, without guilt and remorse.

Has Wanda experienced this abuse? Is Carl now also a victim? The answers to both questions appear to be yes. Historically, the older victim of domestic violence is often not identified in regard to the dynamics of abuse, and is not treated using the knowledge base and array of social, legal, and psychological services now available for both victims and perpetrators of abuse. There is increasing recognition that while men are not frequently victims of domestic violence, this correlation begins to change as the age of the victim increases, retaliation being one cause of the abuse to the male victim.

Harris (1996) describes the absence of research and understanding of domestic violence grown old. In her analysis of theoretical approaches to spousal abuse, the current neglect, potential physical abuse, and violation of rights by Wanda is expressed in the description of the social stress or situational model of spouse abuse. In this model, as stress increases, anger and aggression also increase. Harris' data analysis indicates that for older couples name-calling, nagging, and other verbal abuse provide strong provocations for reducing impulse control and may lead to violence. Wanda's current behavior portrays this pattern.

In present APS practice there is an increasing emphasis on examining the dual issues of elder abuse and domestic violence. In Ohio, new APS staff must receive twelve hours of training in domestic violence during the first twenty-four months of practice, with additional training available on a routine basis. For the APS social worker receiving the assignment of Carl's case, it is quite possible that the information regarding the longstanding abusive pattern in their marriage will be unknown. The early intervention by APS will be to establish whether Carl's care is adequate, whether he is aware of his care plan and in agreement with any changes to it, and whether he has concerns about the care provided by Wanda. Interviews will be conducted with Carl privately. Of critical importance is his mental status regarding his ability to make and carry out his own decisions. There is no indication in the case material that Carl has a diminished or impaired mental capacity. His physician is likely to be asked by the APS social worker to document his evaluation of this capacity. The most likely outcome of this initial intervention is the determination that Carl can make his own decisions, is a very angry man, furious at his loss of control, and in need of an advocate regarding decisions that impact his own care.

The focus will then shift to an understanding of Wanda's capacity as a caregiver. Interviews with Wanda are likely to reveal a person with a history of undiagnosed and longstanding depression, poor self-esteem, and social isolation. In supervisory conferences, there may be discussion regarding Wanda's functioning, examining if she has sufficient impairments to refer her internally and identify her as an APS client as well. The social worker may need the opportunity in discussion with the supervisor to recognize the social worker's own struggle of wanting to only sympathize with Wanda's anger at Carl. They also will discuss the son, his availability, or lack thereof, in regard to the care of his father. Whether Wanda can benefit from counseling, a support group, or increased respite services will be considered in discussions with her. However, the primary focus is on protecting Carl from the potential harm presented by Wanda's now unleashed anger and retaliation. If either Carl or Wanda reveal the pattern of domestic violence in their years of marriage, or the collateral contacts do so, referral of Wanda to a domestic violence support group (rather than a hospice support group, for example) will be made.

The direction and outcome of the APS intervention for Carl will be determined primarily by Carl's wishes, assuming he is a mentally clear and alert person. His decisions regarding his care plan will be communicated and followed; options for greater safety will be considered, including moving him to the inpatient hospice services available locally; and an opportunity to seek counseling for him and his wife will be offered. However, ultimately, the plan will be his to make as an intact adult.

If the case is closed prior to Carl's death, all the parties actively involved in his care will be notified, with the information that the case can be re-opened if allegations of suspected or known harm are present. Also possible is that the case will be closed with Carl still at risk of harm from Wanda, if he is aware of his risks, understands them, and decides that he will not accept any of the APS recommendations for his protection. This outcome will be significantly more complicated if the medical providers decide to withdraw from Carl's care due to the high degree of risk based on the decreased care plan made by Wanda. This potential outcome may provoke at best a renewed consideration by the client of the protective service care plans being offered by APS, or a re-opening of the case at the time of the withdrawal of medical care.

If in fact Carl's mental status is or becomes deteriorated, the options for intervention change dramatically. Unless the issues provoking Wanda's neglect and abuse of her husband have been resolved, an outside party will be sought by the court at the request of APS to manage the care decisions for Carl. Is it possible that the first-time-ever understanding of Wanda's experiences as a victim will provide sufficient support to her that relief to her anger and aggression will occur? Evaluation of her behavior as a caregiver is needed in order to determine if APS would recommend to the court that she be allowed to continue as her husband's caregiver and decision-maker. If Carl's incompetence is the outcome, APS involvement and recommendations will be critical until the decision is made by the Probate Court regarding who is to be his decision-maker. If Wanda is appointed guardian, the court will likely order monitoring of the care plan by APS for three months, with a scheduled follow-up hearing. An optimum outcome is continued involvement by hospice, with both relationship and grief counseling available.

BRENDA AND HARRIET

Caregiver stress is apparent in reading the story of this mother, daughter, and granddaughters. The unraveling of such a fragile care plan seems inevitable: six- and eight-year-olds, responsible after school for a chronically ill, demented, suspicious and anxious grandparent; the primary caregiver, a daughter exhausted as a single parent and without gratification and recognition in her work life, finding her own unmet needs washing over her judgment regarding her mother's care needs. Would a social worker have met this family prior to a referral to APS, potentially offering options and supportive services have prevented this unraveling of care? This is not likely.

Brenda is exhausted, not focused on considering the risks and impact of her decisions regarding her mother, but rather on how to get through today, maybe just this hour of this day. This overwhelming combination of responsibilities is typically carried by families with a history of strength based on love and the hope and intention of giving the right care to the parent in need of help. For many, including Brenda, family caregiving occurs in the absence of outside help to assist with the tasks, either on an informal or agency basis.

As described by Burnstein (1988), even when frustrated, guilty, and isolated family members finally reach out for help, the elderly family member may adamantly refuse to cooperate with "outsiders," resulting in the early closing of the case at a senior service agency. If an agency remains involved in this situation, there is the dilemma of identifying the client (family seeking help? the dependent elder?) and what role self-determination will play. The presence of professional or paraprofessional supportive or home health services can provide the necessary feedback regarding the toll on each family member and the adequacy of the plan for the most vulnerable, which could include the grandchildren. Brenda and Harriet appear to exist in their own small circle of care, with the referral to APS bringing the first intrusion into this world.

APS Intake will receive the referral from the police officer, following the return of Harriet to her home. However, it is important to note that the referral could be missed, if the home and presence of the daughter reassures the officer that this was a one-time slip in an adequate care plan. Hopefully, cross-training between APS and local police will result in a set of questions and observations about the care that would indeed lead to a referral the afternoon of Harriet's wandering. The officer may notice that the daughter had not contacted the police herself, upset by her mother's absence. The facts are that she left her mother alone long enough for her to walk a mile from the home (that it was three hours would probably not be revealed by Brenda), and that it is now time for Brenda to leave for work and two very young granddaughters will be in charge of this upset, confused old woman.

Upon receiving the telephone referral, the APS allegation is identified as neglect by caregiver. The description, even limited to the few known facts, conveys a quality of unintentional harm by an overwhelmed family. The assigned social worker will contact the police officer to discuss any additional observations or police history with this family (no prior involvement with police is the likely answer). Along with the referral information, APS Intake will have made use of public information access and include in the creation of the case file the county auditor's information identifying Harriet as the sole homeowner. The visit to the home in the next day or two is either arranged by the social worker through a telephone call to Brenda to set up an appointment, or unannounced, as a means of seeing a more realistic portrayal of the adequacy of the care plan. At that time, only neglect would be the focus. However, that is likely to change soon.

The first home visit is likely to reveal one of three outcomes: (1) a six-year-old and eight-year-old in charge of a demented grandmother; (2) an exhausted daughter who works the 3:00 p.m. to 11:00 p.m. shift and finds her mother's demanding behaviors difficult; or (3) Harriet alone, the most troubling outcome of all. Additional care and use of available resources are an early focus of discussions with Brenda. Now is the time that Brenda's resistance to using her mother's financial resources for her care would likely become apparent. The additional finding of exploitation will be added to the allegations when the daughter's refusal to use her mother's own money for needed care is clear, and this is likely to become apparent quickly. The interaction between mother and daughter, including the use of threats to place her in a nursing home and locking her in her room or similar outbursts, will add a new allegation: verbal abuse.

An understanding of the burdens of caregiving and the culture of this family will be important tools in the assessment. The information conveys a working class family, probably never or only occasionally on public income benefits due to Harriet's long years of work as a domestic, and proud of the accomplishments of home ownership and savings.

Inquiring about health insurance coverage may reveal that in fact Medicaid is the only resource available to this self-employed woman who may not have ever worked for employers who paid into Social Security for her. The cultural heritage of this family is likely African-American, indicating the importance of honoring the elder member by use of her family name, for example, and recognizing the traditions of family care versus the "easy" use of formal care providers.

Research by Hudson (1994) indicates another complicating characteristic of this cultural background. African-American participants in a study of perceptions of elder abuse rated incidents as more severe than did the white respondents. The research also found that participants with less formal education included a wider range of behaviors as abusive than those with more years of formal education.

Brenda may well feel remorse and guilt over her actions toward her mother, and understand quickly the meaning and purpose of the social worker's visit to the home. She may react with hostility or with a breakdown of tears and acknowledgment of her exhaustion and frustration with her mother. In either case, the social worker must persist with the assessment of the need for protective services. The possible hostility and threat to the social worker's safety will create some delays, a likely return with a co-worker or supervisor, possibly police. In extreme instances, the APS legal counsel may seek a court order to prevent the caregiver from interfering with the investigation and the order issued by the Probate Court will be presented at the home by the social worker and police.

The assessment of Harriet indicates a significantly impaired woman, suffering both physical and mental decline. The medicine bottles with current prescriptions indicates a physician is involved with Harriet and the social worker will contact the doctor to obtain information about the recommended care plan and the evaluation of the client's mental status. If the physician is not familiar with or prepared to complete a formal statement of "Expert Evaluation" for the Probate Court regarding the need for a guardian, referral to a geriatric assessment center will be made, requesting a psychiatric assessment appointment. This will delay the critical documentation regarding Harriet's ability to make her own decisions, but will definitively examine the possibility of a reversible dementia (e.g., untreated thyroid disease).

After a few discussions with Brenda, the social worker understands the history of closeness and the desire to take care of her mother, out of the dual and somewhat contradictory motivations of love and self-preservation for her own family by an inheritance and a home. What explanation is there for the disregard for Harriet's safety and the carelessness and impulsiveness of Brenda's actions? How can Brenda be helped to address the dilemmas regarding the multiple needs of her family?

The APS social worker's primary responsibility is to establish a care plan for Harriet that will ensure her safety. Engaging Brenda in making that plan together, or, if that fails, seeking court orders to impose a plan of protection is a critical APS decision made with supervisory and legal consultation. The principle of seeking the least restrictive outcome will guide the APS case decisions, with the goal of keeping Harriet in her own home as she desires being an optimal outcome. Communicating an understanding of Brenda's experiences as a caregiver is critical in motivating her to cooperate with a more appropriate care plan, likely to include adult day care and the expenditure of some of Harriet's funds.

The concept of "spoiled identity," as presented by nurses Beck and Phillips (1983), may be helpful. This concept was developed to explain the dynamics of the abuse of confused elders by family members. The "spoiled identity" of the demented difficult person, often exhibited in behaviors considered alien to the well-known personality of the person and repugnant to the family, can lead to responses by the family that are outside their usual norms, permitting a reduced sense of responsibility and protection. The outcome of a "spoiled identity" may be a no-win or double-bind situation for families of the confused difficult elderly. They can hang onto the former identity of the person, and experience a continual prolonged grieving, or recognize that the beloved person is not present as in the past. The risk of the second coping mechanism is that it severely diminishes the emotional bonds and increases alienation from the person in need of care. This dilemma is common to the family dynamics of caregiving. Therefore, allowing Brenda to talk about her experiences as a daughter, including her reactions to patients at the nursing home where she works, may help her more objectively recognize her choices and cooperate with a plan for the care of her mother.

A potential outcome for Brenda and Harriet is to open the caregiving arrangements to Harriet's sons, hopefully with additional family members also able to assist, and to recognize that the savings that the matriarch of this family accumulated must now be spent for her care. Preserving the family home for her is important and preserving the family's identity as a loving resource is also important. Providing the grandchildren with less burdensome roles and more control over their disrespectful behavior is an additional goal. Achieving this requires extensive use of community resources, including adult day care and respite sitter services. Some of these services may be available through agencies funded by the Older Americans Act, indicating that there will be no fee structure for services but rather a donation system. This is an optimal outcome for this mother and daughter.

The APS social worker will close Harriet's case when there is an established care plan. Harriet is demented and unable to make her own service arrangements. Securing a safe and stable plan for her is necessary. Those involved in her care will be notified of the case closing, and informed that they can again refer the case to APS Intake if concerns regarding harm to Harriet reoccur.

CONCLUSION

In presenting the social work and specifically the Adult Protective Service response to these three case scenarios, some overall concluding statements are pertinent. Often the point of referral to APS is at a time of crisis, the "train wreck" in the final years of the person's long life. Earlier history and relationships that have had a major impact in shaping these final chapters in a long life are often unknown to APS staff. Action to protect is urgently needed. APS staff typically do not have the luxury of time to understand the dynamics that led to the crisis presented to them. In the broader social work functions in the field of aging there may be ample and rich opportunities for the understanding of the life story that clarifies and explains the scenes now being played out in the final weeks, months, or years of life. The senior center recreation/socialization programs, senior housing sites, nutrition programs, transportation services, adult day care and home health/rehabilitation services, as well as a variety of social service and mental health agencies, may have the staff involvement and time to use reminiscence and individual as well as relationship counseling.

One of the critical functions of collaboration between these community agencies and APS is to provide information that will assist the APS staff in understanding the life history and relationships that impact the current situation that has led to the need for protection. Sharing of information involves issues of confidentiality. However, if the community provider shares the concerns about the allegations of harm, or may in fact be the referral source to APS, there is an appropriate opportunity to share information without the client's written or verbal consent, if it is provided for the purpose of protecting the person from harm. The analysis of these case studies provides an understanding of how this historical information can greatly enhance and clarify the direction that may be most efficient and effective for the protection of the client and the successful provision of services.

This material has been presented in the context of Ohio law, with its particular definitions of abuse, neglect, self-neglect, and exploitation, as well as the particular protocols and practices of one county in Ohio. The need to establish a common taxonomy of terms has been well documented by Hudson (1991, 1994) and others. The wide and troubling variation between state APS laws is a subject of debate and concern. Hopefully, this analysis of case content has presented an understanding of the dynamics of adult protective services that provides the clarity needed for effective social work practice regardless of the specifics of state law.

REFERENCES

Abramson, M. (1985, September). The autonomy-paternalism dilemma in social work practice. *Social Casework: The Journal of Contemporary Social Work,* 387-393.

Beck, C., & Phillips, L. (1983). Abuse of the elderly. *Journal of Gerontological Nursing, 12* (3-4), 98-99.

Bozinovski, S. (1997). Self-neglect among elders: Conceptual framework diagram. *Project Report: National Association of Adult Protective Services Administrators (NAAPSA).*

Brandl, B., & Raymond, J. (1997). Unrecognized elder abuse victims: Older abused women. *Journal of Case Management, 6* (2), 62-67.

Burnstein, B. (1988, October). Involuntary aged clients: Ethical and treatment issues. *Social Casework: The Journal of Contemporary Social Work,* 518-520.

Cook-Daniels, L. (1997). Lesbian, gay, male, bisexual and transgendered elders: Elder abuse and neglect issues. *Journal of Elder Abuse & Neglect, 9* (2), 39-41.

Gruman, C., Stern, A., & Caro, F. (1997). Self-neglect among the elderly: A distinct phenomenon. *Journal of Mental Health and Aging, 3* (3), 309-323.

Harris, S. (1996). For better or for worse: Spouse abuse grown old. *Journal of Elder Abuse & Neglect, 8* (1), 1-5.

Hudson, M. (1991). Elder mistreatment: A taxonomy with definitions by delphi. *Journal of Elder Abuse & Neglect, 3* (2), 1-20.

Hudson, M., & Carlson, J. (1994). Elder abuse: Its meaning to middle-aged older adults–Part 1: Instrument development. *Journal of Elder Abuse & Neglect, 6* (1), 29-54.

Hudson, M. (1994). Elder abuse: Its meaning to middle-aged and older adults–Part 2: Pilot results. *Journal of Elder Abuse & Neglect, 6* (1), 55-81.

Longres, J. (1994). Self-neglect and social control: A modest test of an issue. *Journal of Gerontological Social Work, 22* (3/4), 3-20.

Nelson, G., Eller, A., Streets, D., & Morse, M. (1995). *The field of adult services: Social work practice and administration* (pp. 12-22, 218-225). Washington, DC: NASW Press.

Peach, J., Koob, J., & Kraus, M. (2001). Psychometric evaluation of the Geriatric Depression Scale (GDS): Supporting its use in health care settings. *Clinical Gerontologist, 23* (3/4), 57-68.

Rooney, R. (1992). *Strategies for work with involuntary clients.* New York: Columbia University Press.

Multidisciplinary Teams
in the Clinical Management
of Elder Abuse

Georgia J. Anetzberger, PhD, ACSW
Carol Dayton, MSW, ACSW
Carol A. Miller, MSN, RN, C
John F. McGreevey, Jr., MD
Maria Schimer, JD, MPH, RN

SUMMARY. Multidisciplinary teams (M-teams) promote elder abuse detection and intervention. They vary by auspice, intent, and abuse orientation. However, their benefits, structure, and organization are fairly uniform. This article initially describes and classifies M-teams. Then the five authors of this publication are assembled as a community/consortium elder-specific M-team to collectively analyze the three case studies earlier presented. *[Article copies available for a fee from The Haworth Document Delivery Service: 1-800-HAWORTH. E-mail address: <docdelivery@haworthpress.com> Website: <http://www.HaworthPress.com> © 2005 by The Haworth Press, Inc. All rights reserved.]*

KEYWORDS. Multidisciplinary teams, elder abuse, detection and intervention, case analysis

---

[Haworth co-indexing entry note]: "Multidisciplinary Teams in the Clinical Management of Elder Abuse." Anetzberger, Georgia J. et al. Co-published simultaneously in *Clinical Gerontologist* (The Haworth Press, Inc.) Vol. 28, No. 1/2, 2005, pp. 157-171; and: *The Clinical Management of Elder Abuse* (ed: Georgia J. Anetzberger) The Haworth Press, Inc., 2005, pp. 157-171. Single or multiple copies of this article are available for a fee from The Haworth Document Delivery Service [1-800-HAWORTH, 9:00 a.m. - 5:00 p.m. (EST). E-mail address: docdelivery@haworthpress.com].

Multidisciplinary teams (M-teams) have a long history in addressing elder abuse. The concept seems to have originated over fifty years ago, with the underpinnings of adult protective services. During the 1950s and early 1960s forums were held in communities across the country to discuss the growing number of impaired older adults living alone without nearby family support, potentially at risk of neglect and exploitation (Hall, 1971). The composition of these early forums included many different professional disciplines and service sectors. For example, according to the community planner for one convened by Cleveland's Welfare Federation, the forum's "success lies in bringing to bear the knowledge, leadership, concerns and activities of many different segments of the community . . . multidisciplinary in character" (Barry, 1963: 1). Forum members included social workers, physicians, nurses, attorneys, psychiatrists, educators, agency executives, and court judges.

In addition to their multidisciplinary cooperation, these early forums were characterized by their concern about case situations that reflected complex and difficult human conditions, suggesting social breakdown. Returning to the Cleveland example, the cases discussed by the Welfare Federation had two qualities: (1) "aberrant behavior . . . which manifested itself in ways detrimental to health and safety of self or others, which showed inability to conduct normal activities of daily living," and (2) "a combination of problems which seemed to call for different types of professional help . . . but frequently these problems were . . . of such complexity, responsibility, or long duration as to require more authority or resources than the agencies could provide" (Barry, 1963:4).

DEFINITIONS AND DIMENSIONS

Since their beginnings, multidisciplinary teams have remained an important strategy for elder abuse detection and intervention (Teaster & Nerenberg, 2004). Generally speaking, M-teams are groups of three or more professional disciplines that have been assembled for the purpose of problem identification and treatment recommendation. The wide range of M-teams that exists can be dissected along three dimensions: auspice, intent, and abuse orientation.

With regard to multidisciplinary team auspice, there are two varieties: organization-specific and community/consortium. Organization-specific M-teams emerge from and represent the needs of a particular institutional or agency setting, typically a hospital or an adult protective services agency. Boston's Beth Israel Hospital's elder assessment team illustrates the former. The core group consists of three hospital staff–a clinical social worker, physician, and nurse practitioner, who review referred patients to determine elder abuse and to recommend reporting and treatment (Matlaw & Mayer, 1986; Matlaw & Spence, 1994). Cleveland's Benjamin Rose Community Services elder abuse and ethics case consult team represents the latter. It is composed of staff nurses, social workers, and program administrators, who advise in the handling of the agency's adult protective services cases at the request of their assigned case managers (Nagpaul, 2001).

Community/consortium M-teams are formed by specific communities or geographic regions or by established elder abuse networks. They not only include different professional disciplines, they also have a membership which represents different agencies and service systems. For instance, the M-team for the San Francisco Consortium for the Prevention of Elder Abuse has representatives from nine distinct settings, including mental health, geriatric medicine, law enforcement, and adult protective services (Wolf & Pillemer, 1994). Half of the M-teams in rural Montana developed as a community sought ways to deal with a problem client situation. Core team members represent public service providers–the adult protective services social worker, public health nurse, sheriff, and county attorney (Sekora, 1991). In Cleveland, the Consortium Against Adult Abuse formed a clinical consultation team of select service providers from various disciplines and agencies to review cases referred by Consortium members. The team eventually evolved to develop screening tools, practice guidelines, and even special programs, like a support group for older battered women, based largely upon needs identified through case analysis.

Multidisciplinary teams can have two broad intents: case analysis or education/program planning. All of the M-teams described above provide case analysis, and the Consortium Against Adult Abuse's team evolved to do program planning as well. In offering case analysis, M-teams provide both clinical assessment and suggestions for needed services on referred cases. Again, this is especially valuable in complex elder abuse situations that do not present easy solutions (Mixson et al., 1991). Additionally, community/consortium M-teams can "assist in seeing that services are delivered to clients by all agencies available to meet the need, rather than a single public or private protective services agency" (Bernotavicz, 1982). An M-team formed by New York City's Mount Sinai Medical Center and Victim Services Agency also offered education and program planning. The two agencies collaborated to develop training curricula, protocols, and a resource directory for elder abuse recognition and referral (Mount Sinai/VNS Elder Abuse Project, 1988).

Finally, the abuse orientation of multidisciplinary teams can be either elder abuse-specific or non-elder abuse-specific. Those that are elder abuse-specific can consider either multiple abuse forms or a single abuse form. The M-teams discussed thus far analyze any and all abuse forms referred to them. In contrast, Fiduciary Abuse Specialist Teams (FAST), which originated in California and have gained acceptance elsewhere, narrow their focus to elder financial abuse (Aziz, 2000; Allen, 2000). Non-elder abuse-specific M-teams typically represent established geriatric or ethics groups that have formalized relations with adult protective services and provide case consultation when requested. One example is Denver's Community Bioethics Committee, which was developed to support the local adult protective services program by providing consultation and making recommendations on cases involving incapacitated adults with complex medical and social issues (Otto, 2000). Another example is the collaboration between Baylor College of Medicine and Texas adult protective services. Adult protective services staff are members of the Baylor geriatric assessment team, and as such, participate with the team in its comprehensive assessment and evaluation process (Dyer et al., 1999).

BENEFITS

That multidisciplinary teams have endured so long suggests the important role that they can play in addressing elder abuse. Without focusing on any particular dimension, it can be said that M-teams benefit the abuse detection and intervention process in three ways: (1) They offer a more holistic perspective to the situation of elder abuse than could be offered by any single discipline alone. Combining the orientations, expertises, and philosophies of several disciplines (or systems) is perhaps the best guarantee that all aspects of a situation are assessed and all possible remedies considered. (2) M-teams assure that no single discipline has the sole responsibility for handling complex and challenging elder abuse situations that often seem to defy resolution. Rather, responsibility is shared among multiple disciplines. (3) M-teams help forge relationships among professionals that transcend consideration of individual cases, and serve to promote a community-wide approach to elder abuse prevention and treatment. Although M-teams often emerge from formal elder abuse networks, just as frequently, they help develop or strengthen informal professional ties, which can lead to the establishment of such networks.

STRUCTURE AND ORGANIZATION

Hwalek, Williamson, and Stahl (1991) analyzed rural and urban multidisciplinary teams in Illinois with respect to the roles and responsibilities of team members. They found that regardless of professional discipline, team members uniformly saw themselves as providing advice to persons making case referrals, using the expertise of their professional backgrounds. Likewise, the work context of the teams was similar, consisting typically of two-hour monthly meetings, ongoing consultation as required, use of discussion and reference to professional literature, and keeping meeting minutes. Only the role of the M-team coordinator was unique. That individual was seen as the team leader and took responsibility for arranging and managing team meetings. Furthermore, the coordinator served as liaison between team members, helping to select cases for discussion and providing follow-up activities.

Nerenberg (1991) notes the dynamic process of multidisciplinary teams. They tend to begin small, informal, and unsophisticated. As their skills increase and relationships evolve, M-teams begin to open their meetings to more participants, formalize proceedings, and insure desired competence among team members through newcomer orientation and ongoing education.

Certainly more established multidisciplinary teams are likely to codify their structure and operations. This may include delineating the number of team members, which disciplines or service systems must be represented, and how members are identified and oriented. For example, the Illinois Department on Aging's (1990) *Multidisciplinary Team Member Handbook and Coordinator Guidebook* gives the following membership representation: mental health, medicine, legal, law enforcement, clergy, and financial. Moreover, it states that the elder abuse provider agency appoints the M-team coordinator, who recruits team members. In addition, procedures may be written for completing M-team tasks, and as type and number of cases reviewed at meetings, protections around client confidentiality, and use of team recommendations. The North Carolina Department of Human Resources' (1989) *Guidelines for Development of Adult Protective Services Multidisciplinary Teams* also offers suggestions on such potential issues as resolving conflicts that may arise and establishing trust among members.

REVIEW AND COMMENTS ON THE THREE CASE STUDIES

At its best, clinical management in elder abuse requires both discipline-specific and multidisciplinary team perspectives. Earlier articles in this publication present the former, offering the viewpoints of an attorney, physician, nurse, and social worker in abuse detection and intervention for the three case studies of Jane, Wanda and Carl, and Brenda and Harriet. Here the same four professionals offer an M-team perspective on the same elder abuse situations. To do this the individuals were convened as a group and asked to function as a community/consortium elder abuse-specific M-team engaged in case analysis. They also were given a set of instructions to frame their discussion: (1) Each team member has the profession and job that she or he has in real life. (2) A member of the elder abuse network which serves as auspice to the M-team refers the case for team consideration. The visiting nurse refers Jane, Carl's physician refers Wanda and Carl, and the hospital social worker (based upon the concerns of her colleagues in the emergency department) refers Brenda and Harriet. (3) The information offered by the elder abuse network member seeking team consultation reflects the totality of the case study as originally written, even if it is unlikely that this kind of detail would be known. (4) The M-team has no more than 45 minutes to spend on each of the three case studies. (5) The guest editor of this publication functions as the M-team coordinator, facilitating case assessment and recommendations, guiding group discussion, and recording comments made.

In analyzing the three case studies, the multidisciplinary team was asked minimally to consider four related questions. However, if a specific question did not seem applicable to a given situation, it could be excluded. Likewise, questions could be added in order to better understand and address a case under review. The four general discussion questions follow: (1) Does the situation represent elder abuse? If so: What is the nature of the elder abuse? Is the situation reportable under Ohio's adult protective services law? Are there any reservations in making a report? (2) What are the overriding issues or concerns in this situation? Does anything require urgent attention? (3) Who is the client(s)? What case plans or interventions seem indicated? What challenges might be encountered in case plan implementation or intervening in the situation? (4) What are the probable outcomes in this situation?

Highlights from the multidisciplinary team case analyses are presented below. The three cases are analyzed in the order they were described previously in this publication.

Jane

Attorney: In deciding whether or not Jane's situation is reportable, I first need to go to the statutes and look at the definition of "neglect" in Ohio's adult protective services law. When I do, it seems that Jane falls under that definition as self-neglecting.

Nurse: My biggest concern is for Jane to get a good geriatric assessment. I have a question about whether the visiting nurse has enough evidence to make a report to adult protective services. There are a lot of people out there who are reclusive and perhaps living at some risk, but they're entitled to live the way that they want.

Physician: My understanding is that if you have a suspicion of abuse, neglect, or exploitation, it's appropriate to report. With Jane, there's at least evidence of a safety issue. Reporting may help provide answers to questions surrounding her situation. It is true that a lot of people in health care think that making a referral to adult protective services is like calling in the cops. It's seen as punitive.

Social Worker: I would see the visiting nurse making the report, realizing that she's entered a home where things have been isolated and hidden a long time. Jane's either disinterested or depressed. She doesn't realize the risk that her age and impairments are likely to bring to her living situation over time–the risk of fire because of all the clutter, the risk of further injury–these are all very significant risks. I do understand that people don't like turning someone in to the government, which may come with a heavy hand and say, "You can't live like this. You need to start changing things." That's an unfortunate misrepresentation of what will happen, because the adult protective services social worker will be committed to respecting Jane's right to refuse services, if she has a comprehension of her risk and wants to stay. Because Jane has been so isolated, it may be that no one has made any offer to help. With her history and personality, it may take a while before the visiting nurse, adult protective services social worker, or anyone else melts down her resistance and she accepts help.

Attorney: How far along this road do you go–cajoling, trying, failing?

Social Worker: Not too far, because there are risks of harm that could be life-threatening, and the seriousness of the concerns need to be presented directly to Jane. The required written notice of intent [for an adult protective services investigation in Ohio] given at the first visit with Jane by the adult protective services social worker will do that, some would argue way too early in the effort to help.

Nurse: The sad reality is that how far the visiting nurse can go will be probably 99% determined by Medicare reimbursement requirements.

Physician: Assuming that Jane has decisional capacity, intervention will stand or fall on someone's ability to form an alliance with her, where Jane and a service provider see themselves as working together in removing obstacles to her safety. Of course, the key to successfully working with Jane is gaining her trust, and that means not going into the situation saying, "I know what's best."

Social Worker: In adult protective services, we begin as a neutral party. We try to convey that we neither believe nor disbelieve the report. We take it as a statement of concern. I think of adult protective services as an alarm clock that goes off in people's lives, alerting them that there are sufficient concerns that the government has become involved.

Physician: It would seem that Jane needs to undergo some kind of medical assessment. It may be that she has conditions that, if treated, would dramatically reduce her risks. Also I wouldn't assume that I know for certain that Jane's living where she wants and how she wants. It may be that because she lived at a time when trusting people cost her dearly that shutting everyone off isn't totally a matter of choice. My advice is to focus on Jane's ability to live independently in her current home, to address her medical concerns so that she feels better, and eventually to help her develop some insight about her isolation and its effects. Unless we are faced with overwhelming evidence of risk, where she takes no steps to improve her situation, I think removing her from the home should not be the goal, because she'd be miserable and live a poor quality of life from her perspective.

Nurse: There are two other issues of concern–nutrition and her driving. Both are risks. The visiting nurse should suggest the possibility of meals-on-wheels, meals prepared by a homemaker, or groceries delivered.

Attorney: Jane is so independent that something like taking her license away probably will not stop her from driving. The risk of her driving is great, even on country roads with little traffic.

Social Worker: The adult protective services social worker and visiting nurse should work together, and stay involved. It may take some time before Jane accepts help. What's important is for someone to be around to extend help when she is ready to receive it.

Wanda and Carl

Attorney: Under Ohio's adult protective services law, the definitions of "abuse" and "neglect" seem to apply in this situation.

Social Worker: This case should be reported to adult protective services. Wanda has called the doctor saying that Carl is ending treatment. We know that Carl is a strong-willed, opinionated person. It's unlikely that he's decided to let his wife manage his life. The doctor's only heard from Wanda about ending Carl's treatment. He hasn't heard it from Carl himself. I would think that the doctor knows that Wanda is bitter and withholding adequate care. Therefore, the doctor should be reporting neglect, and perhaps impending abuse. That doesn't preclude being concerned about Wanda, and the fact that she's suffered abuse. But I'm not hearing that Wanda's impaired, and that's a consideration in Ohio's adult protective services law.

Physician: Reporting is important, because Wanda has taken Carl's decision-making away from him for herself. No matter how unsympathetic Carl might be, she doesn't have the right to do that. In addition, there are little things that Wanda is doing that as isolated incidents may pale next to some of the things that Carl has done to her, but they're still not right. Finally, I'd make the report to help

Wanda. She feels trapped, stuck. That's a high-risk caregiving situation. I don't see anything in terms of love and affection between Wanda and Carl to help get through the difficulty of this caregiving. I also struggle about who's the client here. The immediate one is Carl, but Wanda was a victim of abuse for years, and she's still in this difficult situation. Maybe with some help, she can rescue herself.

Nurse: I would advise the doctor to make a referral for a visiting nurse. I think a nurse could get in there, collect more information, relieve some of the caregiving stress, and maybe get some interventions in to help with Carl's care. You could make a justification for skilled nursing and even medical social work under Medicare, but it would probably end up being hospice services. I would like to see the doctor do that as the next step, before reporting to adult protective services.

Attorney: We really don't know whether or not Carl is on more aggressive cancer treatment. We don't know that he hasn't sought out alternative therapies. We don't really know that Carl hasn't said to Wanda that he's sick and tired of going through this. It may be that Wanda is simply acquiescing to Carl's will in telling the doctor to discontinue treatment.

Social Worker: It is not uncommon for victims of domestic violence to fantasize about doing their abuser in. The opportunity to actually fatally harm someone rarely comes along, but when it does, the results can be disastrous. Part of the domestic violence in later life that we see in adult protective services is the retaliation syndrome. Here men die sooner. Women are the caregivers. They're bitter, and they have no outlet for their feelings. One of the outcomes of Wanda's phone call to the doctor is that Wanda will have to live with her guilt if any of her behavior made Carl's suffering greater. It seems to me that the doctor could say to Wanda, "This is a drastic decision. I need to discuss it with Carl. Your son needs to be advised of the decision."

Attorney: Physicians wouldn't necessarily see a phone call about ending treatment as a dramatic event. I have seen in my own life where it's the wife who has the energy to make the call.

Nurse: Also, the wife is power of attorney, and may not view Carl as very competent at this time.

Attorney: A question arises around what treatment they are discontinuing. It's one thing to stop chemotherapy or radiation; it's another thing to stop palliative care.

Physician: I look at the phone call as a trigger for a number of things. First, it's a trigger to sit down and evaluate Carl's treatment to date. There has to be a conversation with Carl to do this. Second, it's a trigger to evaluate Carl's health care wants and needs now. It may be that a visiting nurse or hospice can help. Third, the phone call triggers a consideration of what's best for Wanda. Does she want to stay in the house and be the primary caregiver? If she does, what limits can she set without being neglectful?

Attorney: There are certain legal obligations that you assume as a spouse. On the other hand, if Wanda were to say, "I can't handle this anymore," she would not legally be required to provide care. Slavery went out with the Civil War.

Social Worker: If this came to adult protective services, the case plan is likely to include domestic violence help for Wanda and in-patient hospice for Carl. Will Carl agree to this? The son may help in facilitating intervention. He's escaped the situation, but he's not unaffected by what's happening.

Nurse: There are clearly two victims here. Talking to the physician, I would say, "Wanda may not be your patient, but she has needs, too. She requires help with caregiving." The physician is a major authority figure. He can make sure that services get in and stay in.

Physician: The physician at least can tell Wanda about available services. He also can sit down with Carl and say that Wanda can't handle the caregiving anymore. This may seem paternalistic, even dictatorial, but Wanda may not be enough empowered to make that statement on her own.

Brenda and Harriet

Physician: This case is clear-cut. Harriet is demented and wanders. She's spending significant periods of time at home under the eye of young children. One of her granddaughters is stealing from her. There's also some threat of constraint. There's a lot of evidence here for making a report to adult protective services.

Nurse: Harriet also is probably not getting her medications properly. Her medical care isn't adequate. You even have to wonder if Brenda is buying medications for Harriet, because they're probably expensive.

Attorney: The hospital social worker has a double reporting responsibility here–a report regarding Harriet to adult protective services and one regarding the granddaughters to child protective services.

Social Worker: The police bringing Harriet home would notice that Brenda didn't make the report herself, that she's about to leave for work, that there are children in charge, etc. So we might expect a report from the police as well. It's helpful for adult protective service to have multiple eyes on a situation. If the situation was called into adult protective services, we would open the case on the basis of abuse, neglect, and exploitation–all three. But it's a sympathetic situation. There's lots of indications that this has been a loving family. We have an absolutely exhausted mom, trying to support her family in jobs that don't gratify her. She sounds like she's worried about her kids and losing what had been a supportive relationship with her mother.

Physician: The other thing to deal with is the fact that Brenda is essentially dependent upon Harriet for financial security, or at least for her home. Her reasons for being a caregiver are at least in part financial and so the decisions she makes will be influenced by that fact. If Harriet goes into a nursing facility, Brenda and her children will need to find another place to live.

Attorney: It may be that Harriet needs a guardian, since she has significant cognitive impairment.

Nurse: Brenda has vested interest. Maybe she shouldn't be in charge of decisions about her mom. The local volunteer guardianship program might be a source for a guardian, since Harriet is probably indigent and so qualifies for the program.

Attorney: There's also the issue of Brenda in her employment. You don't know that she won't do at home the kinds of things that she's alleged to have done to nursing facility residents at work. That's a side issue, but it may be evidence of a pattern.

Social Worker: This reminds me of a dilemma that sometimes hits adult protective services social workers. If they're aware that a caregiver may have committed a criminal act, do they report it? Drug dealing is the most common circumstance. For example, the grandson may be providing good care, but he's also dealing in drugs. Do you report him? The outcome is likely that the grandmother will go to a nursing facility without his care. Certainly when we witness a crime, we report it. The dilemma comes when we suspect a crime, but don't know for sure. You may not want to know everything.

Physician: This case is hard in working out a solution, because most of what you do to help Harriet is going to put Brenda and her daughters in a poor situation. This doesn't mean that you don't do it, but here the end may be that a family is out on the streets, homeless, or that Brenda doesn't have her kids anymore.

Attorney: Child day care may be available to Brenda for her daughters, and adult day care for her mother. We all need to get over that if we report these people that their lives will be miserable, because there are interventions which can help.

Nurse: There are so many services available locally that can help in this situation. There are services from the Alzheimer's Association—information and caregiver support groups for Brenda, Safe Return for wanderers like Harriet. There's all the resources available through PASSPORT [Ohio's home and community-based services Medicaid waiver program for impaired older people]. Although there will be a lien placed upon the house as a result of being a PASSPORT client, Brenda could continue living there. Brenda's wrapped up in just surviving, but she might be receptive to help, if it was offered.

Social Worker: I see Brenda as the classic kind of caregiver who's tired. She's just trying to get through the next hour, and she's not seeing the bigger picture. It isn't that she's not smart enough or capable enough. No one is forcing her to see the big picture, and she's too tired to look at it herself. Her brothers need to be pulled in. They need to be asked to share the responsibilities of taking care of Harriet.

REFERENCES

Allen, J.V. (2000). Financial abuse of elders and dependent adults: The FAST (Financial Abuse Specialist Team) approach. *Journal of Elder Abuse & Neglect, 12*(2), 85-91.

Aziz, S.J. (2000). Los Angeles County Fiduciary Abuse Specialist Team: A model for collaboration. *Journal of Elder Abuse & Neglect, 12*(2), 79-83.

Barry, M.C. (1963, March). *Responsibility of the social welfare profession in providing guardianship and protective services.* Paper presented at the Arden House Seminar on Protective Services for Older People, Harriman, NY.

Bernotavicz, F. (1982). *Improving protective services for older Americans: A national guide series: Community role.* Portland, ME: University of Southern Maine, Human Services Development Institute.

Dyer, C.B., Gleason, M.S., Murphy, K.P., Pavlik, V.N., Portal, B., Regev, T. & Hyman, D.J. (1999). Treating elder neglect: Collaboration between a geriatrics assessment team and adult protective services. *Southern Medical Journal, 92*(2), 242-244.

Hall, G.H. (1971). Protective services for adults. In R. Morris (Ed.), *Encyclopedia of social work: Vol. 2* (pp. 999-1007). Washington, DC: National Association of Social Workers.

Hwalek, M., Williamson, D., & Stahl, C. (1991). Community-based M-Team roles: A job analysis. *Journal of Elder Abuse & Neglect, 3*(3), 45-62.

Illinois Department of Aging. (1990). *Multidisciplinary team member handbook and coordinator guidebook.* Springfield, IL: Author.

Matlaw, J.R., & Mayer, J.B. (1986). Elder abuse: Ethical and practical dilemmas for social work. *Health and Social Work, 11*(2), 85-98.

Matlaw, J.R., & Spence, D.M. (1994). The hospital elder assessment team: A protocol for suspected cases of elder abuse and neglect. *Journal of Elder Abuse & Neglect, 6*(2), 23-37.

Mixson, P., Chelucci, K., Heisler, C., Overman, W., Sripada, P., & Yates, P. (1991). The case of Mrs. M.–A multidisciplinary team staffing. *Journal of Elder Abuse & Neglect, 3*(4), 41-55.

Mount Sinai/VSA elder abuse project. (1988, October). *Aging Network News, 5*(6), 1, 20.

Nagpaul, K. (2001). Elder abuse and ethics case consult team at the Benjamin Rose Institute. *OCAPS Newsletter, 2*(2), 3-4.

Nerenberg, L. (1991). The San Francisco Consortium Multidisciplinary Team: Another perspective. *Journal of Elder Abuse & Neglect, 3*(3), 66-71.

North Carolina Department of Human Resources. (1989). *Guidelines for development of adult protective services multidisciplinary teams.* Raleigh, NC: Author.

Otto, J.M. (2000, March/April). Bioethics committee aids APS workers in making complex medical decisions for incapacitated adults. *Victimization of the Elderly and Disabled, 2*(6), 89, 94.

Sekora, D. (1991). The Montana adult protective services teams: A rural perspective. *Journal of Elder Abuse & Neglect, 3*(3), 62-66.

Teaster, P.B. & Nerenberg, L. (2004). A national look at elder abuse multidisciplinary teams. Washington, DC: National Committee for the Prevention of Elder Abuse.

Wolf, R.S., & Pillemer, K. (1994). What's new in elder abuse programming? Four bright ideas. *The Gerontologist, 34*(1), 126-129.

Index

BOOK ORDER FORM!

Order a copy of this book with this form or online at:
http://www.haworthpress.com/store/product.asp?sku=5018

The Clinical Management of Elder Abuse

___ in softbound at $24.95 (ISBN: 0-7890-1947-7)
___ in hardbound at $39.95 (ISBN: 0-7890-1946-9)

COST OF BOOKS _____

POSTAGE & HANDLING _____
US: $4.00 for first book & $1.50
for each additional book
Outside US: $5.00 for first book
& $2.00 for each additional book.

SUBTOTAL _____

In Canada: add 7% GST. _____

STATE TAX _____
CA, IL, IN, MN, NY, OH & SD residents
please add appropriate local sales tax.

FINAL TOTAL _____
If paying in Canadian funds, convert
using the current exchange rate,
UNESCO coupons welcome.

❑ BILL ME LATER:
Bill-me option is good on US/Canada/
Mexico orders only; not good to jobbers,
wholesalers, or subscription agencies.

❑ Signature _____

❑ Payment Enclosed: $ _____

❑ PLEASE CHARGE TO MY CREDIT CARD:
❑ Visa ❑ MasterCard ❑ AmEx ❑ Discover
❑ Diner's Club ❑ Eurocard ❑ JCB

Account # _____

Exp Date _____

Signature _____
(Prices in US dollars and subject to change without notice.)

PLEASE PRINT ALL INFORMATION OR ATTACH YOUR BUSINESS CARD

Name

Address

City   State/Province   Zip/Postal Code

Country

Tel   Fax

E-Mail

May we use your e-mail address for confirmations and other types of information? ❑ Yes ❑ No We appreciate receiving your e-mail address. Haworth would like to e-mail special discount offers to you, as a preferred customer.
We will never share, rent, or exchange your e-mail address. We regard such actions as an invasion of your privacy.

Order From Your **Local Bookstore** or Directly From
The Haworth Press, Inc. 10 Alice Street, Binghamton, New York 13904-1580 • USA
Call Our toll-free number (1-800-429-6784) / Outside US/Canada: (607) 722-5857
Fax: 1-800-895-0582 / Outside US/Canada: (607) 771-0012
E-mail your order to us: orders@haworthpress.com

For orders outside US and Canada, you may wish to order through your local
sales representative, distributor, or bookseller.
For information, see http://haworthpress.com/distributors

(Discounts are available for individual orders in US and Canada only, not booksellers/distributors.)

Please photocopy this form for your personal use.
www.HaworthPress.com

BOF04